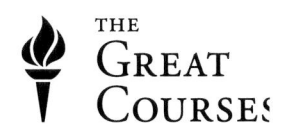

The Science of Integrative Medicine

Brent A. Bauer, M.D.
Mayo Clinic

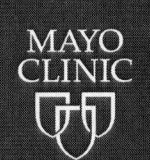

PUBLISHED BY:

THE GREAT COURSES
Corporate Headquarters
4840 Westfields Boulevard, Suite 500
Chantilly, Virginia 20151-2299
Phone: 1-800-832-2412
Fax: 703-378-3819
www.thegreatcourses.com

Copyright © The Teaching Company, 2016

Printed in the United States of America

This book is in copyright. All rights reserved.

Without limiting the rights under copyright reserved above,
no part of this publication may be reproduced, stored in
or introduced into a retrieval system, or transmitted,
in any form, or by any means (electronic, mechanical,
photocopying, recording, or otherwise),
without the prior written permission of
The Teaching Company.

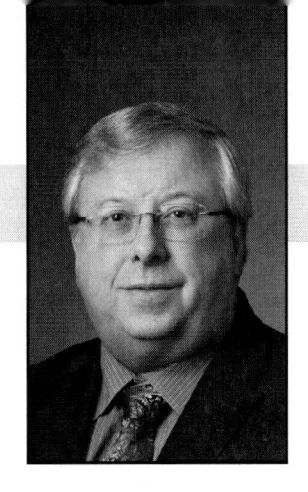

Brent A. Bauer, M.D.

Professor of Medicine
Director of the Complementary and
Integrative Medicine Program
Mayo Clinic

Brent A. Bauer, M.D., is board certified in internal medicine and is a Professor of Medicine and the Director of the Complementary and Integrative Medicine Program at Mayo Clinic, where he has been on staff for 24 years. His main research interest has been the scientific evaluation of integrative medicine therapies, which patients and consumers are using with increasing frequency. Dr. Bauer has authored several book chapters and more than 100 papers on this topic and is the medical editor of *Mayo Clinic Book of Alternative Medicine*. He is a member of numerous scientific review panels and is currently collaborating on more than 20 Mayo Clinic studies that evaluate integrative medicine therapies, ranging from acupuncture to valerian. He is the medical director of Rejuvenate, the first spa at Mayo Clinic. He is also the medical director of the Well Living Lab, a collaboration between Delos, a company that specializes in what's called wellness real estate, and the Mayo Clinic Center for Innovation. Dr. Bauer's work is at the forefront of the emerging field of integrative medicine, which combines the best of conventional medicine with the best of evidence-based complementary therapies. ■

About Mayo Clinic

Mayo Clinic is a nonprofit organization committed to providing expert, whole-person care to everyone who needs healing. The Mayo Clinic mission is to inspire hope and contribute to health and well-being by providing the best care to every patient through integrated clinical practice, education, and research. For more information, visit www.mayoclinic.org/about-mayo-clinic or http://newsnetwork.mayoclinic.org/.

At the turn of the 20th century, Dr. Charlie and Dr. Will Mayo organized medical professionals in a new way to better care for patients. They created a system that allowed doctors to take the time to thoroughly investigate patient problems and to quickly and easily get help from other specialists.

The system was built on the idea that two heads are better than one. It also encouraged a continual search for better ways of diagnosis and treatment.

Through growth and change, Mayo Clinic remains committed to its heritage: thorough diagnosis, accurate answers, and effective treatment through the application of collective wisdom to the problems of each patient. ■

Table of Contents

Introduction
Professor Biography i
About Mayo Clinic.. ii
Integrative Medicine and Your Wellness... 1

Lecture Guides

Lecture 1
    Complementary and Integrative Medicine................................3

Lecture 2
    Making the Case for Integrative Medicine..............................25

Lecture 3
    Herbal Supplements...46

Lecture 4
    Supplements in Practice...68

Lecture 5
    Mind-Body Medicine...90

Lecture 6
    Guided Imagery, Hypnosis, and Spirituality........................... 112

Lecture 7
    Practicing Meditation 136

Lecture 8
    Moving Meditation: Yoga, Tai Chi, and Qi Gong....................157

Lecture 9
    Relaxation Therapies 181

Table of Contents

Lecture 10
    Effective Acupuncture 203

Lecture 11
    Massage Therapy and Spinal Manipulation 225

Lecture 12
    Living Well 249

Supplemental Material

Bibliography 272
Image Credits 288

Disclaimer

This series of lectures is intended to increase your understanding of how doctors diagnose and treat diseases and how you can improve your own health by being an active and informed patient. However, these lectures are not designed for use as medical references to diagnose, treat, or prevent medical illnesses or trauma, and neither The Teaching Company nor the lecturer is responsible for your use of this educational material or its consequences. Furthermore, participating in this course does not create a doctor-patient relationship. The information contained in these lectures is not intended to dictate what constitutes reasonable, appropriate, or best care for any given health issue, nor does it take into account the unique circumstances that define the health issues of the viewer. If you have questions about the diagnosis, treatment, or prevention of a medical condition or illness, you should consult your personal physician. The opinions and positions provided in these lectures reflect the opinions and positions of the relevant lecturer and do not necessarily reflect the opinions or positions of The Teaching Company or its affiliates.

The Teaching Company expressly DISCLAIMS LIABILITY for any DIRECT, INDIRECT, INCIDENTAL, SPECIAL, OR CONSEQUENTIAL DAMAGES OR LOST PROFITS that result directly or indirectly from the use of these lectures. In states that do not allow some or all of the above limitations of liability, liability shall be limited to the greatest extent allowed by law. ■

Integrative Medicine and Your Wellness

Close your eyes for a moment and imagine what your best version of yourself looks like. What picture would you paint of yourself? Do you feel full of energy? Are you having fun? Are you enjoying spending time with the people around you? These are just a few examples of ways you may describe what you'd ideally like your life to look like—and your overall wellness plays a large role in helping you achieve that vision.

Achieving overall wellness, especially in this day and age, is no simple feat. Conventional Western medicine, as good as it is, doesn't have cures for all that ails us—especially many of the often-chronic conditions that plague people today, such as arthritis, back pain, neck pain, fibromyalgia, and anxiety.

Whether you're looking for help managing a chronic condition or searching for new ways to improve your wellness and live a healthier, more enjoyable life, integrative medicine may be the complement to conventional medicine that you're looking for.

In this course, you'll learn first about what constitutes a foundation for good health, which rests on four key practices: nutrition, exercise, stress management, and a strong support network (NESS). These components are the basis for a healthy life, so you'll be reminded of them often throughout the course. In addition, you'll learn about the 10 most promising practices in integrative medicine—treatments that you might consider as part of your own health and wellness practice.

• Acupuncture	• Music therapy
• Guided imagery	• Spinal manipulation
• Hypnotherapy	• Spirituality
• Massage	• Tai chi
• Meditation (both stationary and movement-based)	• Yoga

In addition to exploring each of these practices, you'll also delve into other areas of integrative medicine, including relaxation therapies, other mind-body techniques, herbal medicine, and dietary supplements. You'll learn about what scientific research says about the safety and effectiveness of these practices, as well as how to integrate them safely into your own life. In addition, you'll get an inside look at how Mayo Clinic incorporates these techniques into its own practice—for its patients, their families, and its employees. You'll also learn how to find and use credible scientific research to help guide your choices. Throughout this course, you'll be exposed to integrative medicine and even receive instruction on some practices you can do at home right away.

By the end of this course, you should have a good idea of what you can do each day to improve your wellness. Although your personal wellness plan starts with a foundation for good health (NESS), you also may begin to identify integrative practices that can support your own personal wellness and help you lead a healthier, happier life. ■

Lecture 1

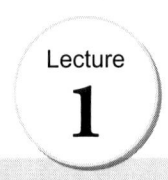

Complementary and Integrative Medicine

If you're taking this course, you might have heard about how natural or holistic practices are being used to complement conventional medicine. You might be interested in learning how to integrate these practices effectively into your life, or—if you're skeptical—you might be wondering if there's any scientific basis for alternative medicine. This course strives to answer your questions and concerns about this type of medicine. In this lecture, you will be introduced to complementary and integrative medicine.

An Inexpensive Way to Reverse Aging

- In 2013, Dean Ornish, M.D., and his colleagues published a remarkable study. They worked with men in their 50s and 60s who had a nonaggressive form of prostate cancer for which the men did not receive medical treatment—no surgery, no chemotherapy.

- Dr. Ornish brought the men in for training on how to eat a healthy diet. They were also given guidance on exercise. They received training in different stress management techniques, such as yoga and meditation, and were instructed to practice them 60 minutes a day. Finally, he had the men come in once a week to participate in a support group.

- The men in this study followed a comprehensive lifestyle approach consisting of four main components: nutrition, exercise, stress management, and social support (NESS).

    ○ For nutrition, this study followed a low-fat diet that emphasized whole grains, fruits, and vegetables, similar to the popular

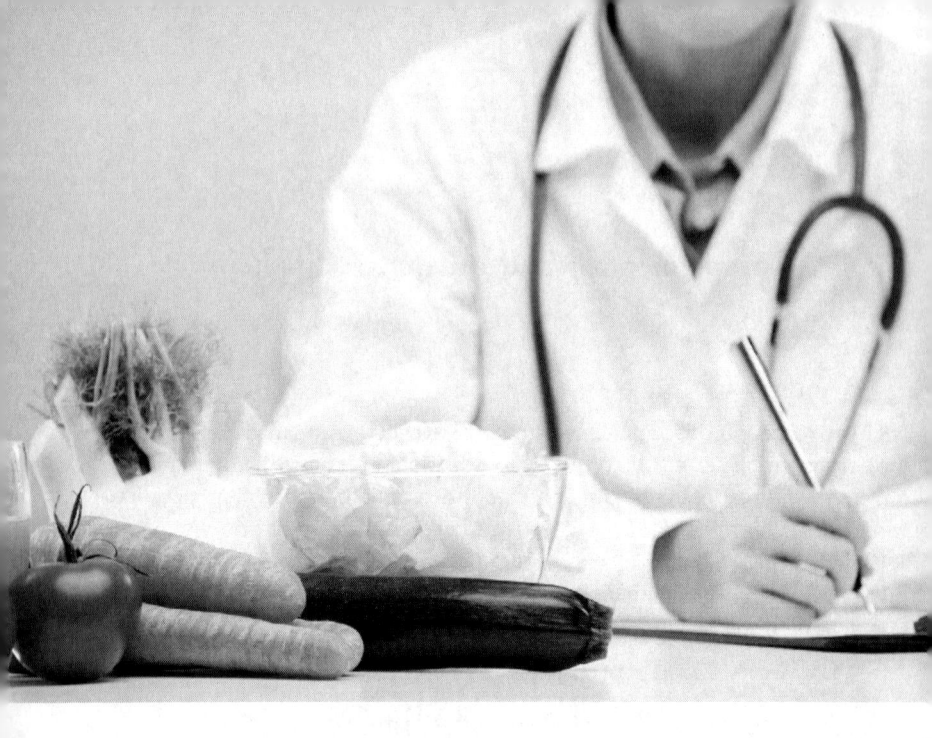

Mediterranean or DASH diets. Both of these diets have been shown to lower the risk of heart disease and high blood pressure.

- For exercise, the men were asked to take part in 30 minutes a day of walking or another form of moderate exercise, such as swimming or biking. They did this almost every day—six days a week.

- They also practiced some form of stress management, such as yoga or meditation, for 60 minutes a day, almost every day.

- The study supplied the final component of the comprehensive lifestyle approach—a strong support system—with a weekly one-hour support group. There are significant benefits of friendship on mental, emotional, and physical health for both men and women.

- At the beginning of the study and again after five years, Dr. Ornish measured the men's telomeres, which are the protective caps on the ends of the arms of chromosomes. Our chromosomes contain our DNA and are what allow us to replicate ourselves. As the telomeres shrink, our DNA can be exposed and damaged, leading to aging and increasing the risk of cancer, heart disease, osteoporosis, and other diseases that are associated with aging.

- After three months, Dr. Ornish was able to detect a significant improvement in telomerase, the enzyme that makes telomeres, which was a good sign that he was on the right track. He then followed these men for five more years. He found that the men who didn't follow the comprehensive lifestyle approach had further shortening of their telomeres, the expected result as people age. However, those who continued to engage in the comprehensive lifestyle approach saw their telomeres lengthen.

- The comprehensive lifestyle approach appears to not only slow the aging process, but to some extent, it also seems to reverse it. More studies are needed, and some are already underway, but scientists believe that increases in telomere length may help prevent a variety of chronic illnesses and maybe even lengthen lifespan.

- If you're interested in improving your health, many complementary medicine practices can help. Not only can they speed your recovery from illness or surgery, but they can also help you cope with a chronic condition. Complementary practices, such as meditation and yoga, can work to keep you healthy and may prevent many diseases.

Integrative Medicine

- It wasn't that long ago that complementary medicine was considered "unorthodox" or "alternative" medicine and largely shunned by most physicians. But over time, people continued to experiment with alternative practices, such as massage, acupuncture, and meditation.

- In the last 20 years, there has been a change in attitude toward alternative medical treatments, accompanied by an evolution in terminology. In the 1990s, the terms "unorthodox" and "alternative" were replaced with the term "complementary and alternative medicine" (CAM), which became an umbrella term for everything from herbal remedies to mind-body therapies to traditional Chinese medicine.

- Attitudes changed first among patients and consumers, and in recent years, we've seen continued growth in the interest and in the use of many alternative therapies by patients and consumers. A number of surveys looking at the use of CAM by adults in the United States suggest that more than a third of Americans are already using CAM practices as part of their health care.

- With the most advanced medical technology in the world, why are Americans turning to complementary and alternative treatments?

    o Patients in general are taking a greater role in their own health care. Thanks largely to the Internet, today's typical patient is more aware of health issues and is more open to trying different treatment approaches.

    o Adults in the baby-boom generation don't like getting older or the effects of aging, and they're open to a variety of treatments. Many people prefer to try complementary methods before taking a pharmaceutical approach.

    o There is a large degree of chronic stress in the American lifestyle, including job hassles, marital conflict, and financial worries. Complementary medicine has several highly effective, evidence-based approaches to dealing with stress that don't involve drugs.

- In parallel with this growing interest in alternative medicine, a tremendous amount of research has been done in recent years on alternative therapies. In the process, this research is helping to identify many genuinely beneficial treatments.

- As evidence concerning the safety and efficacy of many of these therapies grows, physicians are starting to integrate aspects of complementary medicine into conventional medical care. This has led to the current term "integrative medicine." The idea is not to replace conventional medicine but to find ways to complement existing treatments.

- Recently, more scientific studies on alternative treatments are being conducted, giving physicians more confidence in recommending certain therapies. In addition, the doctor-patient relationship has changed significantly in recent years—it's more of a partnership. Furthermore, there has been a shift of focus toward wellness and preventive medicine in medicine today, and this is where complementary practices can play a huge role.

- Most likely, medical practitioners will gradually become more open to the idea of integrative medicine. It is much more accepted now as part of medical treatment, both in the medical world and by Western culture in general. But keep in mind that it's not a replacement for conventional medicine.

- Currently, there are 65 academic medical centers that are part of an organization called the Academic Consortium for Integrative Medicine & Health. It's clear that complementary medicine is not a fad, and many academic medical centers are taking steps to better understand unconventional treatments to be aware of their safety and effectiveness.

- This does not mean that all complementary treatments are okay to use. Doctors should not prescribe complementary therapies without having some reason to believe that they work, and some therapies carry significant risks. But it does mean that certain therapies have merit and should be discussed with your doctor to see if they can aid in health and healing.

Talk with Your Doctor

- Your doctor can help you think through a number of issues surrounding complementary medicine, including the following.
    - Point out whether the treatment has any potentially dangerous side effects.
    - Help you determine the correct dosage of a particular supplement.
    - Give you advice on which therapies might be the most appropriate for you.
    - Let you know if a product you're taking may interact with a medication you currently use.
    - Put you in touch with someone who performs a particular therapy or who can teach you how to do it.

Working with Your Doctor

- If your doctor has never mentioned practices such as acupuncture or massage, you might be nervous about bringing them up. You might worry that your doctor will be too quick to reject the idea or that you'll be criticized or told to stop a treatment that you feel is helping you.

- Before we judge doctors too quickly, we have to recognize that many patients have been harmed—in some cases, even killed—by unethical and immoral products that have been touted online and in various stores as miracle cures. Unfortunately, some products have turned out to be tainted with either pharmaceutical drugs or herbs that are dangerous and that caused a host of other problems.

- It's understandable why some doctors who have seen this type of harm might be averse to unconventional therapies. If your doctor happens to fall into this category, recognize that he or she may have had an unfortunate past experience with a patient that has produced skepticism.

- Before talking with your doctor, make sure to do your homework and make it known that you're not looking for a miracle cure. Instead, you're looking for evidence-based complementary practices that you can incorporate with your conventional care.

- If your doctor still isn't comfortable about discussing dietary supplements or acupuncture with you, ask for a referral to someone who may be able to help you, such as a pharmacist or a specialist in a particular field.

- Even if they may be skeptical, most doctors are aware that unconventional therapies are very popular. And it's important that they know what you're taking or practicing to be sure that the therapy is safe for you. Make sure that you understand the potential risks as well as benefits.

The 10 Most Promising Practices in Integrative Medicine

- The following is a list of 10 treatments that you might consider as part of your health and wellness practice.

    1. **Acupuncture** is a Chinese practice that involves inserting very thin needles at strategic points on the body and is commonly used for nausea and fibromyalgia and to treat many kinds of pain.

    2. **Guided Imagery** (sometimes called visualization) involves bringing to mind a specific image or series of memories to produce certain responses in the body. It's used to treat headaches and some forms of pain.

3. **Hypnosis** involves a trancelike state where the mind is more open to suggestion. It may be used to help manage pain, anxiety, and tension headaches.

4. **Massage** comes in many different varieties, and some have specific health goals. It can address pain, anxiety, and fibromyalgia.

5. **Meditation** involves clearing and calming the mind by focusing on your breathing or a word, phrase, or sound. It is used to help treat anxiety, stress, and high blood pressure.

6. **Music therapy** can influence both your mental and physical health. It may help patients with Alzheimer's disease and autism, as well as depression.

7. **Spinal manipulation** (also called spinal adjustment) is practiced by chiropractors and physical therapists. It's particularly helpful for low-back pain.

8. **Spirituality** is focused on an individual's connection to others and to the search for meaning in life. These connections help people deal with medical illness and chronic disease.

9. **Tai chi** is a graceful exercise in which you move from pose to pose. It's been shown to improve balance and flexibility.

10. **Yoga** involves a series of postures that often includes a focus on breathing. It is commonly practiced to relieve stress, as well as treat heart disease and depression.

Suggested Reading

Bauer, "Chinese Medicine and Integrative Medicine in the United States."

Hensrud, *The Mayo Clinic Diet*.

———, *The Mayo Clinic Diet Journal*.

Hensrud, et al, *The New Mayo Clinic Cookbook*.

McGarey, *Physician within You*.

Ornish, *Dr. Dean Ornish's Program for Reversing Heart Disease*.

Pang, et al, "Complementary and Integrative Medicine at Mayo Clinic."

Wahner-Roedler, et al, "Physicians' Attitudes toward Complementary and Alternative Medicine and Their Knowledge of Specific Therapies: A Survey at an Academic Medical Center."

Wahner-Roedler, et al, "Physicians' Attitudes toward Complementary and Alternative Medicine and Their Knowledge of Specific Therapies: 8-Year Follow-Up at an Academic Medical Center."

Lecture 1 Transcript

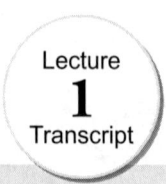

Complementary and Integrative Medicine

What if I told you there was a therapy that could reverse aging and potentially prevent cancer, and that this therapy was relatively inexpensive and had no side effects? Would you be interested? What if I told you that this therapy involved nothing but nutrition, exercise, stress management, and a strong support system? What if I told you that this approach has been shown to improve your cells at the genetic level? Sound too good to be true?

Hello, I'm Doctor Brent Bauer, director of Mayo Clinic's Complementary and Integrative Medicine Program. If you're taking this course, you've probably heard about how natural or holistic practices are being used to complement conventional medicine. You may be interested in learning how to integrate these practices effectively into your own life, or if you're skeptical, you may be wondering if there's any scientific basis for alternative medicine or if it's all just a bunch of hooey.

I hope to answer your questions and concerns about alternative medicine in the course of these lectures. But first, let's begin by exploring that therapy I just mentioned—the inexpensive way to reverse aging.

In 2013, Dr. Dean Ornish and his colleagues published a remarkable study. They worked with men in their 50s and 60s who had a non-aggressive form of prostate cancer for which the men did not receive medical treatment—no surgery, no chemotherapy. I think this is an important group because if these men weren't young, healthy subjects, in which case the results might not mean as much to people who are older or who are facing a diagnosis of cancer or another serious disease.

Dr. Ornish brought the men in for training on how to eat a healthy diet. They were also given guidance on exercise. They received training in different stress management techniques, such as yoga and meditation, and were instructed to practice them 60 minutes a day. Finally, he had the men come in once a week to participate in a support group.

Let's take a closer look at the comprehensive lifestyle approach the men followed in the Ornish study. They followed four main components, which we can remember with the mnemonic N-E-S-S, or NESS, like Eliot Ness, or the Loch Ness monster—nutrition, exercise, stress management, and support.

For nutrition, the Ornish study followed a low-fat diet that emphasized whole grains, fruits, and vegetables, similar to the popular Mediterranean or DASH diets. Both of those diets have been shown to lower the risk of heart disease and high blood pressure. A new variation on these diets, called the MIND diet, has also been shown to significantly reduce the risk of late-onset Alzheimer's disease. We'll talk about that diet at more length in the next lecture, but you probably already know that your health can benefit from including more fruits and vegetables in your diet, as well as more whole grains and fish, and consuming less fat and sugar.

The second component of the Ornish lifestyle approach was exercise or fitness. Contrary to what you may be thinking, that didn't mean pumping iron or running marathons. The men were asked to take part in 30 minutes a day of walking or another form of moderate exercise, such as swimming or biking. But they did it almost every day, six days a week.

Third was some form of stress management, such as yoga or meditation, which they practiced for 60 minutes a day—again, almost every day. For many of us who pride ourselves on being insanely busy, that may sound like a lot of time away from our smartphones. But if you consider that stress is probably shortening your life by several years, not to mention reducing the quality of what's left of your life, 60 minutes a day of thoughtful attention to your mind and body starts to sound like a wise investment.

The fourth component was one that is actually lacking in many men's lives—a strong support system. Although some men aren't aware of the importance of social support, there are significant benefits of friendship on mental, emotional, and physical health for everyone—men and women alike. The Ornish study supplied this component of the comprehensive lifestyle approach with a weekly one-hour support group.

At the beginning of the study and again after five years, Dr. Ornish did something very strategic: He measured the men's telomeres. Telomeres are the caps on the ends of the arms of chromosomes. If you remember taking high school biology, you'll recall that you have 23 chromosomes from your mother and 23 from your father. Our chromosomes contain our DNA and are what allow us to replicate ourselves over and over. The Nobel Prize in Physiology or Medicine in 2009 was awarded to researchers who discovered that the telomeres act like a protective cap on the ends of the chromosome arms.

A simple analogy for telomeres is the cap on our shoelaces. When the cap comes off, the shoelace frays, gets shorter and shorter, and no longer works as well. Something similar happens with the chromosomes: as the telomeres shrink, our DNA can be exposed and damaged, leading to aging and increasing the risk of cancer, heart disease, osteoporosis, and other diseases associated with aging.

After three months, Dr. Ornish was able to detect a significant improvement in telomerase. This is the enzyme that makes telomeres, so it was a good sign that he was on the right track. He then followed these men for five more years. He found that men who didn't follow the comprehensive lifestyle approach had further shortening of their telomeres, the expected result as people age. However, those who continued to engage in the comprehensive lifestyle approach saw their telomeres actually lengthen.

This is an amazing result. The comprehensive lifestyle approach appears to not only slow the aging process, but to some extent, also seems to reverse it. More studies are needed, of course, and some are already underway, but scientists believe that increases in telomere length may help to prevent a variety of chronic illnesses and maybe even lengthen lifespan.

Does this mean that following this approach will bring the Fountain of Youth, or prevent everyone from getting cancer? The answer, of course, is no. But I do think it provides a roadmap for experiencing optimal health at any age and regardless of your physical challenges.

If you're interested in improving your health, many complementary medicine practices can help. In fact, some of them were used in the Ornish study. Not only can they speed your recovery from illness or surgery, but they can also help you cope with a chronic condition. Best of all, complementary practices, such as meditation and yoga, can work to keep you healthy and may actually prevent many diseases.

But is complementary medicine real medicine? Is it evidence-based? You may be wondering, "Why is Mayo Clinic, one of the premiere centers of conventional medicine, incorporating acupuncture, massage, and meditation into patient care?" After all, it wasn't that long ago that these types of treatments were considered unorthodox or alternative medicine and largely shunned by most physicians.

At their worst, unorthodox treatments can be dangerous, especially when seriously ill patients abandon conventional medicine for some quack remedy that promises miracles it can't deliver. Like some disreputable bad guy, this kind of alternative medicine could take your money and your life.

But over time, people continued to experiment with alternative practices like massage, acupuncture, and meditation. At first, Western doctors didn't know what to make of these practices. They just weren't part of their medical vocabulary. They didn't know if such treatments were actually helpful or if they might interfere with conventional treatment.

Doctors also weren't used to patients being involved in medical decisions. There was a time not that long ago when the patient met with the doctor and did what the doctor ordered without any questioning.

So when a patient brought up something like hypnosis as a way to try and stop smoking, doctors often dismissed it as junk science and not something worth considering. Acupuncture was viewed as something not much different from voodoo—sticking pins in humans instead of dolls. Herbal remedies were dismissed as the equivalent of snake oil. Patients often felt like they were being punished or ridiculed for bringing up such ideas.

But in the last 20 years, there's been a change in attitude toward alternative medical treatments, accompanied by an evolution in terminology. In the 1990s, the terms unorthodox and alternative were replaced with the term complementary and alternative medicine, or CAM. CAM became an umbrella term for everything from herbal remedies to mind-body therapies to traditional Chinese medicine.

Attitudes changed first among patients and consumers. In spite of general disapproval from the medical establishment, people kept experimenting and trying new approaches to health, often influenced by the medical practices of other cultures. In recent years, we've seen continued growth in interest and in the use of many alternative therapies by patients and consumers. A number of surveys looking at the use of CAM by adults in the United States suggest that more than a third of Americans are already using CAM practices as part of their health care.

With the most advanced technology in the world, why are Americans turning to complementary and alternative treatments? There are actually several reasons.

One is that patients, in general, are taking a greater role in their own health care. Today's typical patient is more aware of health issues and is more open to trying different treatment approaches. The Internet has played a huge role in improving patient education. Two decades ago, patients had little access to research or reliable medical information. Things like clinical trials and pharmaceutical developments were just not available for public knowledge.

These days, however, patients who have, say, arthritis can find a lot of information about it on the Internet. They may find good research that glucosamine, for example, helps with joint pain and doesn't appear to have a lot of risks associated with it. And then they feel empowered to ask their doctor if something like glucosamine might work with their current medication plan.

A second reason for the wider acceptance of complementary treatments is the influence of the baby-boomer generation. This is a group that's not aging quietly into the night. They don't like getting older, or the effects of aging, and they're open to a variety of treatments. As they age, baby boomers are also likely dealing with more medical issues—weight control, joint issues, high blood pressure, and elevated cholesterol. Not everyone wants to take a pharmaceutical approach right off the bat; many prefer to try complementary methods first.

A third reason is the degree of chronic stress in the American lifestyle. Job hassles, commuting woes, marital conflict, financial worries—the list, unfortunately, goes on. Western medicine has excellent medications for short-term stress, but over the long term, those very medications can become just as damaging and even as life-threatening as the stress itself. Complementary medicine, on the other hand, has several highly effective, evidence-based approaches to dealing with stress that involve no drugs at all. Many otherwise healthy people are learning to manage the stress in their lives successfully by using methods like yoga, meditation, massage, and guided imagery.

When you consider that many people, while they're still healthy, are already engaging in such practices, it isn't such a stretch to think that they're turning to complementary treatments when they get sick too. Meditation, for example, can help a person manage the anxiety and discomfort of medical procedures. Massage has been shown to improve recovery rates for patients who've undergone heart surgery, something I'll talk more about in a later lecture. And gentle tai chi or yoga can assist the transition back to an active life after illness or surgery.

Conventional medicine, as good as it is, doesn't have cures for everything. Many people with arthritis, back pain, neck pain, fibromyalgia, and anxiety look to alternative treatments to help them manage these often chronic conditions without the need for strong medications that may have serious side effects, or that may be addictive.

In parallel with this growing interest in alternative medicine, a tremendous amount of research has been done in recent years on alternative therapies, attempting to separate the wheat from the chaff. In the process, this research is helping to identify many genuinely beneficial treatments. So both patient interest and scientific research have caused modern medicine to take a fresh look at these approaches.

As evidence concerning the safety and efficacy of many of these therapies grows, physicians are starting to integrate aspects of complementary medicine into conventional care. This has led to the current term integrative medicine.

Integrative medicine is simply the practice of using conventional medicine alongside evidence-based complementary treatments. Prescribed medications might not completely help a headache or relieve chronic pain, but adding massage, meditation, or acupuncture might be just the extra boost the patient needs. The idea is not to replace conventional medicine but to find ways to complement existing treatments. Integrating the best of both worlds for the optimal benefit of the individual patient—that is how I view integrative medicine.

At Mayo Clinic, the goal for physicians is to provide the best possible care to all our patients. To do this, we often need to evaluate and incorporate the best treatments from all sources.

For example, I can help many of my patients who have arthritis by prescribing anti-inflammatory medications or physical therapy, but it's rare that I can actually cure arthritis. So it's not surprising to me that many of my patients who have to deal with chronic symptoms look to other possible treatments. When I began to see some people benefiting from therapies such as acupuncture, I wanted to learn more. That led me on a journey of exploration I've been on for the past 20 years—a journey that's led me to my current position as Director of the Integrative Medicine Program at Mayo Clinic.

A lot has changed in those 20 years. For one thing, more scientific studies on alternative treatments are being conducted, giving physicians more confidence in recommending certain therapies. Now, if we want to know more about a certain therapy or if our patients have questions, we can look at data in peer-reviewed studies. For example, if someone comes to me and has a question about supplements that are safe to take with high blood pressure, I can look at more than 2,000 different studies, and that can help lead to an informed decision.

Another thing that's changed significantly in recent years is the doctor-patient relationship. Today, it's more of a partnership. Because patients are more educated and ask more questions, doctors need to be open to different ways of thinking and to treatments that might not always follow conventional practices. Instead of dismissing patient questions and ideas, the doctor works with the patient to determine the best course of action.

A third difference in medicine today is the shift of focus toward wellness. This is where complementary practices can play a huge role. Conventional medicine is good for fixing what's broken, but it's not always as useful for preventing future problems. Managing stress, eating healthy, getting plenty of exercise—those actions can help prevent that heart attack from happening in the first place. Complementary medicine can help you reduce stress, eat well, and develop gentle stretching routines to improve balance and muscle tone.

I expect that medical practitioners will gradually become more open to the idea of integrative medicine. When you look at medical students today, they're following natural diets and eating organic foods. Their parents are doing tai chi. These students have yoga sessions before a class, and they meditate together.

That's why it's much more common today to see a doctor prescribing fish oil to lower high triglycerides or suggesting a yoga class to address flexibility issues or stress management. People use complementary practices to treat a variety of diseases and conditions, from preventing a cold to controlling headaches to helping them get a good night's sleep. Overwhelmingly, though, the most common reason people turn to non-conventional treatments is pain—particularly back pain, as well as neck and joint pain.

Integrative medicine is much more accepted now as part of medical treatment, both in the medical world and by Western culture in general. In fact, complementary medicine has become part of our cultural model. But we have to remember that it's not a replacement for conventional medicine. If you have a heart attack, you don't want your doctor chanting over you. You want a heart catheterization procedure to relieve the blockage, and possibly a stent inserted in the damaged artery. You may even need surgery. However, you may find that your recovery can be aided by practicing relaxation exercises such as deep breathing or by being visited by a friendly dog and its owner from a pet therapy program like the one we have at Mayo Clinic.

Currently, there are 65 academic medical centers—places that do research as well as practice medicine—that are part of an organization called The Academic Consortium for Integrative Medicine & Health. It's clear that complementary medicine is not a fad, and many academic medical centers are taking steps to better understand unconventional treatments to be aware of their safety and effectiveness.

Does that mean all complementary treatments are okay to use? No. At Mayo Clinic, we don't prescribe complementary therapies without having some reason to believe that they work.

We approach natural supplements and complementary therapies in the same way we approach conventional medication—if it's strong enough to help us, it's strong enough to hurt us. We've seen people harmed by taking things they shouldn't have. Some therapies carry significant risks, and we'll talk about those later in the course.

It does mean that certain therapies have merit and should be discussed with your doctor to see if they can aid in health and healing.

So how do you work with your doctor? If your doctor has never mentioned practices such as acupuncture or massage, you might be nervous about bringing them up. You might worry that your doctor will be too quick to reject the idea or that you'll be criticized or told to stop a treatment that you feel is helping you.

Before we judge the doctors too quickly, we have to recognize that many patients have been harmed, in some cases even killed, by unethical and immoral products that have been touted online and in various stores as miracle cures. Unfortunately, some products have turned out to be tainted with either pharmaceutical drugs or herbs that are dangerous and that caused a host of other problems.

It's heart-wrenching for a doctor, or any health professional, to see a young woman who has easily treatable breast cancer turn away from conventional medicine because she's been told of the horrors of chemotherapy, only to work with an alternative healer who uses herbs to treat the cancer. That same woman may return to the doctor's office six months later with a much more advanced breast cancer that now requires a greater amount of surgery and chemotherapy, or worse yet, is no longer treatable.

It's understandable why some doctors who have seen this type of harm might be adverse to unconventional therapies. If your doctor happens to fall into this category, recognize that he or she may have had an unfortunate past experience with a patient that has produced this skepticism.

So before talking with your doctor, make sure to do your homework and make it known that you're not looking for a miracle cure. Instead, you're looking for evidence-based complementary practices that you can incorporate with your conventional care. The more evidence there is to support a particular practice—like taking glucosamine for arthritis—the more comfortable doctors feel in recommending it.

If your doctor still isn't comfortable discussing dietary supplements or acupuncture with you, ask for a referral to someone who may be able to help you, such as a pharmacist or a specialist in a certain field.

Even if they may be skeptical, most doctors are aware that unconventional therapies are very popular. And it's important that they know what you're taking or practicing to be sure that the therapy is safe for you. In the case of supplements, sometimes, because people see the word natural on the product, they simply assume it's safe and don't feel the need to discuss it with their doctor.

Remember, if the treatment is strong enough to help you, it's also powerful enough to harm you, or in some cases even kill you. So don't be persuaded by advertisements or claims that the product is all-natural and, therefore, safe. Make sure you understand the potential risks as well as benefits.

As I mentioned earlier, some supplements have reached the market in an adulterated state, containing herbs or chemicals that don't belong in them. In one famous but tragic case, some young women who were going to a weight-loss clinic suddenly developed kidney failure. Many of these women ended up in dialysis or needed kidney transplantation. An investigation found that the clinic was using a Chinese herb, but had inadvertently switched the usual product to one that was very toxic to the kidneys. Compounding this problem, it turns out this particular herb also increases the risk of cancer, and many of these women went on to develop cancer of the urinary tract.

So it's a good idea to talk with your doctor. Your doctor can help you think through a number of issues. For example, your doctor can point out whether the treatment has any potentially dangerous side effects; your doctor can help you determine the correct dosage of a particular supplement; your doctor can give you advice on what therapies might be the most appropriate for you. Not everyone responds the same to every therapy. Meditation might work well for some people, but not for others. Your doctor can let you know if a product you're taking may interact with a medication you currently use. Your doctor can put you in touch with someone who performs a particular therapy or can teach you how to do it. Many academic research centers have meditation, yoga, and nutrition programs on their own.

So what are some of the most promising practices in complementary medicine? Here's a list of 10 treatments that you might consider as part of your own health and wellness practice. We'll spend more time expanding on each of these therapies later in the series, but here is a quick rundown, listed in alphabetical order:

Acupuncture is a Chinese practice that involves inserting very thin needles at strategic points on the body. It's commonly used for nausea, fibromyalgia, and to treat many kinds of pain.

Guided imagery, which is sometimes called visualization, involves bringing to mind a specific image or a series of memories to produce certain responses in the body. It's used to treat headaches and some forms of pain.

Hypnosis involves a trance-like state where the mind is more open to suggestion. Hypnosis may be used to help manage pain, anxiety, and tension headaches.

You likely know what massage is. There are many different kinds of massage, and some have specific health goals in mind. Massage can address pain, anxiety, and fibromyalgia.

The practice of meditation involves clearing and calming the mind by focusing on your breathing or a word, phrase, or sound. Meditation is used to help treat anxiety, stress, and high blood pressure.

Music therapy can influence both your mental and physical health. It may help patients with Alzheimer's disease and autism, as well as depression.

Spinal manipulation, which is also called spinal adjustment, is practiced by chiropractors and physical therapists. It's particularly helpful for low-back pain.

Spirituality has many definitions, but its focus is on an individual's connection to others and to the search for meaning in life. We find that these connections help people deal with medical illness and chronic disease.

Tai chi is a graceful exercise in which you move from pose to pose. It's been shown to improve balance and flexibility

And finally, yoga. Yoga involves a series of postures that often include a focus on breathing. Yoga is commonly practiced to relieve stress, as well as treat heart disease and depression.

In this course, we'll also be talking about a variety of herbs, vitamins, and other dietary supplements. You'll learn what the research tells us about how safe they are and whether or not they can help manage certain conditions

But before you start adding pills, ointments, and extracts to your wellness routine, think back on that study by Dean Ornish and the NESS acronym. The basic components of a healthy life are nutrition, exercise, stress management, and a strong support network. If you smoke cigarettes, eat junk food, and sit around watching television all the time, you can take ginseng and fish oil until the cows come home, but you still won't be healthy.

On this journey to improve your health, and possibly increase your lifespan, start with the basics. Try eating less fast food and more fruits and vegetables. Relax with a warm bath or a few minutes of quiet reflection. Go for a daily walk around the neighborhood. And get together with friends you can enjoy and really talk to. If the Ornish study is right, your cells may start getting younger, so don't be surprised if you start feeling that way too.

Lecture 2

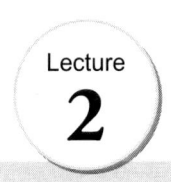

Making the Case for Integrative Medicine

Integrative medicine isn't just about fixing things when they're broken; it's about keeping things from breaking in the first place. It's about preventive medicine and treating the whole person. And in many cases, it means trying new therapies and approaches, such as meditation and tai chi. In this lecture, you will learn about what caring for the whole person means. You will learn some simple, evidence-based ways that you can improve your personal health and overall well-being—through good nutrition, exercise, relaxation, and sleep.

Nutrition

- The Mediterranean and DASH (which stands for "dietary approaches to stop hypertension") diets are your best insurance against high cholesterol, high blood pressure, and heart disease. Their emphasis on whole grains, fruits and vegetables, nuts, olive oil, fish, and poultry offer plenty of variety in a diet intended not necessarily to lose weight—although that may be a side benefit—but to improve your lifelong eating habits.

- The two diets are quite similar, although the DASH diet places more emphasis on lowering your sodium intake and on portion control. Neither the Mediterranean diet nor the DASH diet bans sweets, red meat, or alcohol, but limits them to small amounts.

- These diets have been proven to reduce your risk of heart disease, as well as diabetes and some types of cancer. If strictly followed, they may even help prevent or slow the progression of Alzheimer's disease.

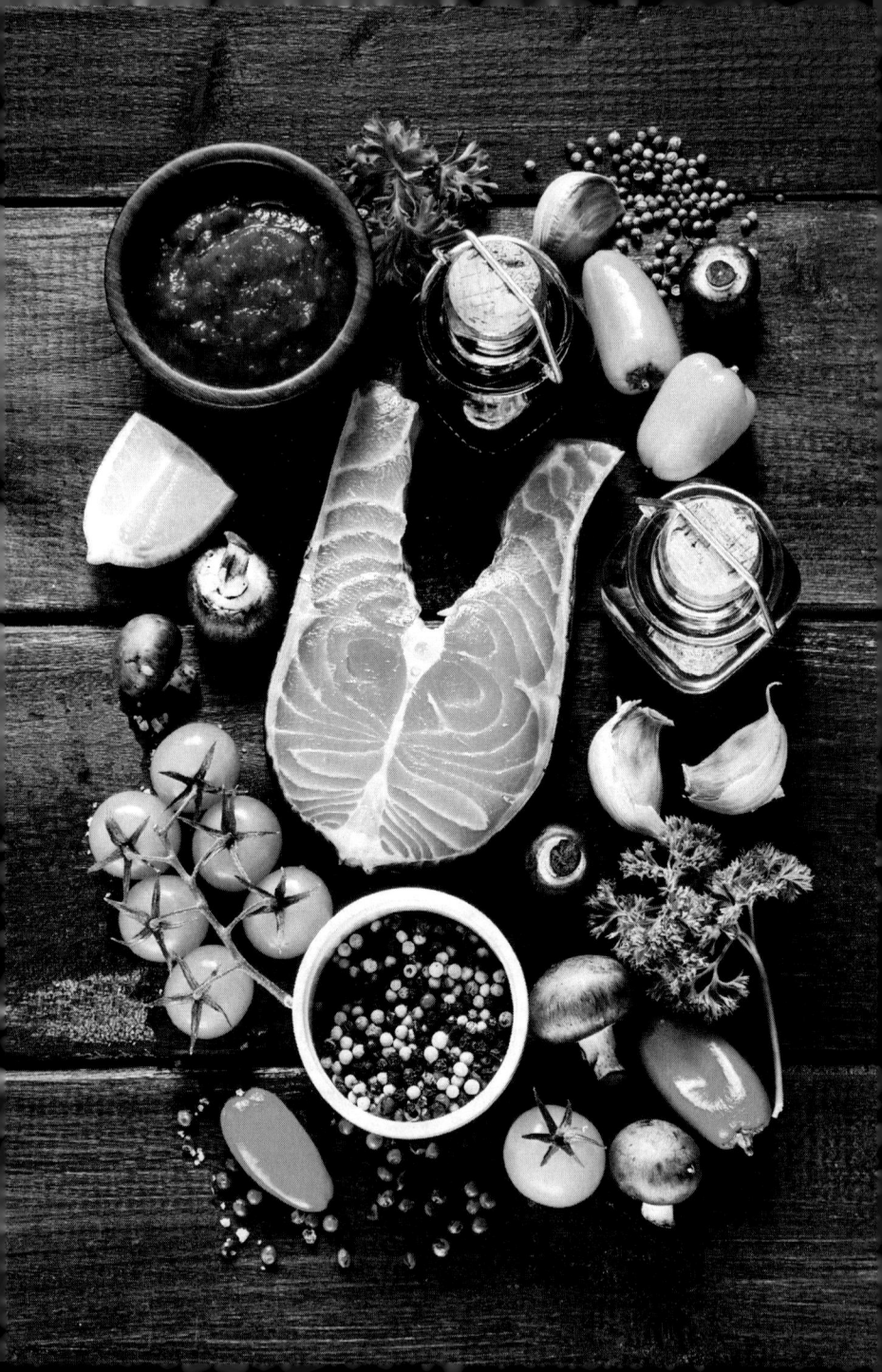

- The Mediterranean and DASH diets have been scientifically proven to be the best diets to achieve long-term health and wellness. Epidemiological and observational studies have shown that these diets reduce the risk of stroke, heart disease, and dementia.

- In a study published in 2015, Rush University Medical Center came out with a new diet called the MIND (which stands for "Mediterranean-DASH intervention for neurodegenerative delay) diet. It's based on the Mediterranean and DASH diets, but it focuses specifically on brain health. Ten brain-healthy foods—including vegetables, nuts, and whole grains—were recommended, and five not-so-brain-healthy foods—including red meats, cheese, and fried food—were restricted.

- The study followed more than 900 people between the ages of 58 and 98 for four and a half years and found that close adherence to the MIND diet in this population reduced the incidence of Alzheimer's disease by 50 percent. Even moderate adherence to the diet reduced the risk by 35 percent, whereas moderate adherence to the Mediterranean and DASH diets showed no such benefit.

- In addition to considering what's on our plates, it's also important to think about how we eat what's on our plates. Many people eat while doing something else—for example, watching television or browsing the Internet. We don't really pay attention to what we're eating, and we eat very quickly.

- Mindfulness means different things to different people, but the traditional concept is about being present in the moment. If you're eating mindfully, then you take your time eating and become fully aware of the tastes and textures of the food in your mouth. This process slows you down.

- If we eat quickly, our bodies don't have a chance to tell us when we're full, so we're overfull before we know it. If you're fully experiencing what you're eating, you might be satisfied with less food.

Exercise

- There are some really great health benefits to exercise. Several studies have shown that aerobic exercise, such as walking, bicycling, swimming, and dancing, reduce age-related brain shrinkage while improving memory and other cognitive functions.

- Exercise also strengthens your cardiovascular and respiratory systems and reduces the buildup of harmful deposits in your arteries by increasing the concentration of high-density lipoprotein (HDL), or "good cholesterol," in your blood. It strengthens your heart so that it can pump blood more efficiently. And that reduces the risk of developing high blood pressure.

- Exercise keeps bones and muscles strong by maintaining bone density, which plays several roles in preventing osteoporosis. And it helps manage your weight, improving diseases and conditions associated with being overweight, such as diabetes. Exercise appears to reduce your risk of certain cancers, including colon, prostate, breast, and uterine lining cancers.

- Exercise also helps you sleep better. Moderate exercise at least three hours before bedtime can help you relax and sleep better at night. A good night's sleep helps maintain your physical and mental health.

- Although researchers say that larger studies are needed to confirm these findings, some research shows that moderate aerobic exercise may help prevent the common cold. Those who have found that exercise does help suggest that it has a positive effect on the cells that impact your immune system.

- There are also psychological benefits to exercise. Exercise raises endorphins, which gives you energy, and increases serotonin, which helps you sleep better. Exercise also brings a sense of accomplishment when you increase your physical ability. Furthermore, exercise enhances the power of connection; many fitness activities and sports involve other people. Exercise can also be a spiritual experience, particularly if you're doing something in nature.

Stress

- A big part of what makes our modern lifestyle so unhealthy revolves around stress. We're too stressed to eat properly, get enough sleep, and find time to exercise. And when we eat too much and sleep too little and don't exercise at all, we become even more stressed. And the more we go around on that vicious cycle, the harder it is to get off.

- No one can avoid stress altogether, but how you manage it is critical to your health and well-being. And there are many complementary practices that can help you do that.

- We have stress responses and relaxation responses. The stress response is the so-called fight-or-flight response. If you are about to get hit by a car, your body automatically increases your heart rate and the blood flow to your muscles, while shutting off the blood flow to less vital body functions, so that you can jump out of the way.

- But most of the stresses we face today don't require a fight-or-flight response. For example, if your boss dumps three extra things on your desk, increasing your heart rate isn't going to help you deal with this kind of stress—yet we use that same stress response.

- And this response becomes our default pathway. It sends out adrenaline day after day, increasing our heart rate. It suppresses our immune system and increases inflammation, all of which lead to problems if they occur all the time for a long time.

- For most people, relaxation takes effort. You have to practice creating the relaxation response—essentially the exact opposite of what happens in the stress response. Most people are so overwhelmed that they have to take a formal approach, such as practicing meditation or deep breathing, to see their heart rate come down, their breathing slow, and their brains begin to focus on the present moment.

- There's a tremendous amount of research on stress and how it impacts people's lives. The stressful situations we experience have a cumulative effect on the body and produce many negative consequences.

- Stress increases inflammation throughout your body, which creates a cascade effect that can lead to a variety of chronic diseases, including heart disorders and stomach problems. Stress can also affect the immune system by producing the hormone cortisol, which increases your susceptibility to colds and flu. Stress also decreases wound healing. Studies have shown that stress may worsen asthma symptoms, skin disorders, chronic pain, and depression.

Rest and Relaxation

- Rest and relaxation are the best antidotes to stress, and they're as fundamental to your health as physical activity and a nutritious diet. They both help slow your heart rate so that your heart doesn't have to work as hard. Relaxation lowers blood pressure and increases blood flow to your major muscles. Regular, deep sleep can improve immune function and reduce signs and symptoms of illness, such as headaches, nausea, diarrhea, and pain.

- A good night's sleep gives you more energy and improves your concentration during the day. It can also help you lose weight. When we're tired, we tend to eat more high-calorie foods to keep our energy up. When we're well rested, we don't need those calories to stay alert.

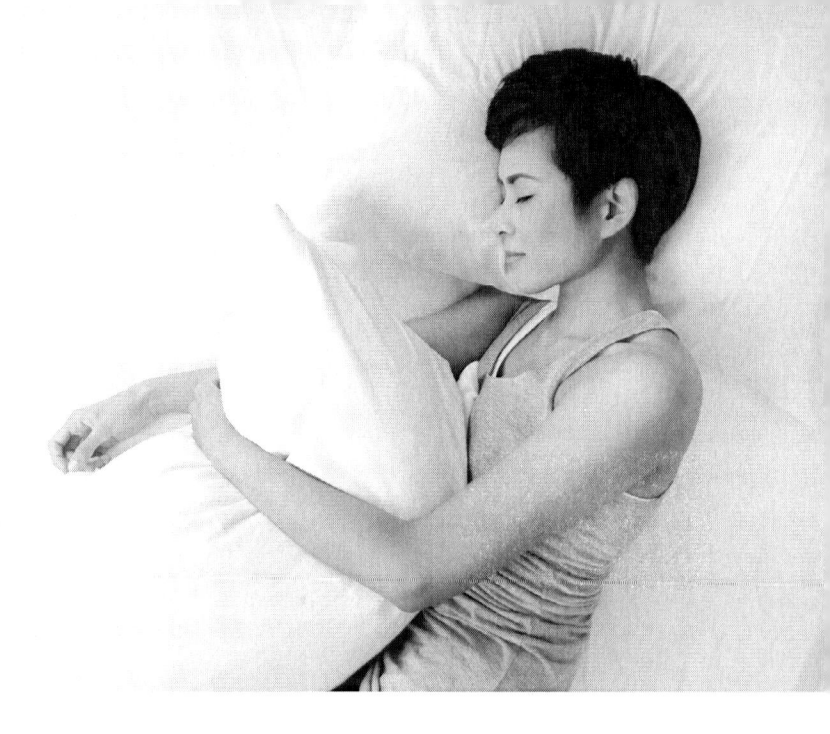

- Most people need seven to eight hours of sleep a night. If you have trouble sleeping or if you just want to improve how well you sleep, some simple changes in your daily routine may help.

    - Develop and stick to a sleep routine. Reading a book is how many people lull themselves to sleep. Some gentle tai chi may help you relax. Turn off the television and all other electronic devices about an hour before bed.

    - Cut down on caffeine, especially in the hours before bedtime.

    - Avoid alcohol and nicotine before bedtime, too; they both interfere with healthy sleep. If you're bothered by heartburn, don't eat for a few hours before you lie down.

- Avoid "trying to sleep" or worrying about not getting enough sleep; doing so is likely to keep you awake. And don't keep checking the clock to see how late it is. Hide your alarm clock in a drawer or turn it away from you if you find yourself looking at it too often.

- Although there are both prescription and nonprescription medications to help you sleep, they generally aren't recommended for long-term use. There are many complementary treatments for insomnia.

- Melatonin is a hormone produced naturally in the brain, and melatonin supplements are widely used for jet lag and sometimes to help people sleep. Melatonin is widely considered safe, but it may cause clotting problems in people taking blood thinners. Also, don't take it if you're pregnant or trying to become pregnant.

- The plant-based supplement valerian may help you get to sleep faster and improve sleep quality. Valerian is also used for anxiety. Discuss valerian with your doctor before trying it. Some people who have used high doses or used it for a long time may have increased their risk of liver damage, although it's not clear if valerian caused the damage.

- Acupuncture and hypnosis are also commonly used to help with insomnia, although research is unclear about their value. Some people say that the smell of lavender helps put them in a peaceful frame of mind, too.

- Don't ignore sleep problems that persist. People with chronic insomnia are more likely to develop psychiatric problems, such as depression and anxiety disorders. Long-term sleep deprivation can also increase the severity of chronic disease, such as high blood pressure and diabetes.

Suggested Reading

Barton, et al, "The Use of Valeriana Officinalis (Valerian) in Improving Sleep."

Centers for Disease Control and Prevention, "Sleep and Sleep Disorders."

Dahm and Smith, *Mayo Clinic Fitness for EveryBody.*

DiFiore, "Diet May Help Prevent Alzheimer's."

———, "New MIND Diet May Significantly Protect against Alzheimer's Disease."

Hensrud, *The Mayo Clinic Diet.*

———, *The Mayo Clinic Diet Journal.*

Hensrud, et al, *The New Mayo Clinic Cookbook.*

Kiecolt-Glaser, et al, "Hostile Marital Interactions, Proinflammatory Cytokine Production, and Wound Healing."

Morris, "MIND Diet Associated with Reduced Incidence of Alzheimer's Disease."

Salter and Brownie, "Treating Primary Insomnia."

Schmidt and Bland, *Brain-Building Nutrition.*

Song, et al, "The Role of Multiple Negative Social Relationships."

Sood, *The Mayo Clinic Guide to Stress-Free Living.*

Wolever and Reardon, *The Mindful Diet.*

World Health Organization, "Spending on Health."

Lecture 2 Transcript

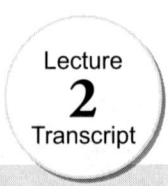

Making the Case for Integrative Medicine

Compared to other countries, the United States spends a lot on health care. In a 2012 study of 34 developed countries, the United States spent just over $8,300 per person, per year, on health care. That's two-and-a-half times greater than the amount spent in other countries. Compared to Norway, which ranks second in health care costs, the U.S. spends an additional $2,500 more per person, per year, on health care. That's a big difference. Yet we have the highest level of obesity, the ninth lowest life expectancy of any major developed country. Where have we gone wrong? Let me count the ways.

We are a country addicted to fried and fatty fast food. It used to be that families got together at the end of the day for a home-cooked dinner. Now we're all so busy, we don't have time for that; we're in convenience mode. Almost half of Americans eat some type of fast food several times a week. Is it any wonder that ½ of Americans are either overweight or obese?

The scary thing is because so many of us are overweight, fat is beginning to look like the new normal. And if people see being fat as normal, they may be less motivated to lose weight. Social norms may be changing, but the dangers of obesity are not. Obesity puts you at serious risk for diabetes, high blood pressure, heart disease, certain types of cancer, sleep apnea, and osteoarthritis.

People who are overweight also are less likely to exercise. According to research published in 2014 by the Centers for Disease Control and Prevention, 80% of Americans fail to get even the minimum amount of exercise needed for a healthy lifestyle. At minimum, it's important to get at least 150 minutes a week of aerobic physical activity, 75 minutes a week of vigorous activity, or a combination of the two. Minimum physical activity guidelines also include doing activities that strengthen all of your major muscle groups at least twice a week. Too little physical activity can lead to obesity, high blood pressure, heart disease, diabetes, and depression, among other health-related issues.

Our sedentary lifestyle is literally killing us. Add up the time you sit at your desk at work, the hours you sit in a car commuting, the time you sit on the couch watching TV, and the hours you sit in front of your home computer, checking email and Facebook and playing video games. The average American spends 13 hours a day sitting down, often getting up only to get something to eat.

And our kids aren't doing much better. Children and teens aged 18 and younger spend 2–3 hours a day in front of the TV, and 2 more hours playing video games or on the computer—and that's outside of schoolwork. Only 1/4 of teens get enough exercise each day.

Scientists have only recently realized how dangerous this sedentary lifestyle is to our health. Inactivity contributes to heart disease, diabetes, cancer, obesity; I think you can finish that sentence yourself by now. In a recent mega-study following over 300,000 people for 12 years, simple inactivity was associated with twice the death rate as obesity alone.

And by the way, in case you hadn't noticed, we're not sleeping very well either. According to the Centers for Disease Control and Prevention, one in four Americans doesn't get enough sleep, leading to, yes, all of those illnesses previously mentioned, and an increase in motor vehicle accidents as well.

I'm betting that not one thing I've said so far has surprised you. We all know that we're not eating right, we're not getting enough exercise, we're spending too much time with TV, computers, and smartphones, and we're not sleeping well. Yes, we know that.

If we're paying attention to life at all, we also know what it takes to eat better, to become more physically active, and to sleep better. This information is in magazines, on TV talk shows, and all over the Internet. You'd have to live under a rock to miss it. We know how to live better.

So why don't we do it? That's the million-dollar question—or maybe the trillion-dollar question if we consider the health-related costs of not doing it. The fact is, we're in trouble with our current health care system; we need to look differently and innovatively at our health strategies.

And this is where integrative medicine can help. Integrative medicine isn't just about fixing things when they're broken; it's about keeping things from breaking in the first place. It's about preventive medicine and about treating the whole person. And in many cases, it means bringing new therapies and approaches to the table—like meditation and tai chi. Sometimes, these integrative approaches are the door openers that help lead people into a complete lifestyle of wellness. Let's take a step-by-step look at what caring for the whole person means.

To begin, let's take a look at some simple, evidence-based ways you can improve your personal health and overall well-being. We'll start with nutrition. We've known for some time now that the Mediterranean diet and DASH diet—which stands for Dietary Approaches to Stop Hypertension—are your best insurance against high cholesterol, high blood pressure, and heart disease. Their emphasis on whole grains, fruits and vegetables, nuts, olive oil, fish and poultry offer plenty of variety in a diet intended not so much to lose weight—though that may be a side benefit—but to improve your life-long eating habits.

The two diets are quite similar, although the DASH diet places more emphasis on lowering your sodium intake and on portion control. Neither the Mediterranean diet nor the DASH diet bans sweets, red meat, or alcohol altogether, but limits them to small amounts. These diets have been proven in study after study to reduce your risk of heart disease, as well as diabetes and some types of cancer. If strictly followed, they may even help prevent or slow the progression of Alzheimer's disease. The Mediterranean and DASH diets have been scientifically proven to be the best diets to achieve long-term health and wellness. Epidemiological and observational studies have shown that these diets reduce the risk of stroke, heart disease, and dementia.

In a study published in 2015, Rush University Medical Center came out with a new diet called the MIND diet. It's based on the Mediterranean and DASH diet, but it focuses specifically on brain health. MIND stands for Mediterranean-DASH Intervention for Neurodegenerative Delay. Ten brain-healthy foods were recommended, and five not-so-brain-healthy foods were restricted. The 10 brain-healthy food groups included: green leafy vegetables—a salad every day; other vegetables; nuts, every other day or so; berries—blueberries especially, but also strawberries; beans, every other day or so; whole grains, at least three servings a day; fish, at least once a week; poultry; olive oil; and wine, one 5-ounce glass a day.

The five unhealthy groups were red meats, less than a serving a week; butter and stick margarine, less than a tablespoon a day; cheese, less than a serving a week; pastries and sweets, less than a serving a week; fried or fast food, less than a serving a week for each.

The study followed more than 900 people between the ages of 58 and 98 for four and a half years, and the results were impressive. Close adherence to the MIND diet in this population reduced the incidence of Alzheimer's by a full 50%. Even moderate adherence to the diet reduced the risk by 35%, whereas moderate adherence to the Mediterranean and DASH diets showed no such benefit.

Obviously, more research needs to be done, but you don't need to wait for the results to improve your own diet. Tape a list of the 15 healthy and not-so-healthy foods to your refrigerator door and start making changes where you can. The truth is, you probably can't do it all, and you can't do it perfectly. But small changes over time can make a difference.

We've talked a lot about what's on our plates. But it's also important to talk about how we eat what's on our plate. Many of us eat while doing something else—watching television, reading a book, on the computer. We eat while we're at our desks in the office or in the car on the way to work. We don't really pay attention to what we're eating, and we eat really quickly.

Mindfulness means different things to different people, but the traditional concept is about being present in the moment. If you're eating chocolate-covered peanuts and not really paying attention, if you're thinking about who you yelled at this morning or what you're going to do tomorrow, that's not eating mindfully, and you'll probably eat a lot more than you intended.

If you're eating mindfully, then you take your time eating and become fully aware of the tastes and the textures of the food in your mouth. This process slows you down. We know that if we eat quickly, our bodies don't have a chance to tell us when we're full, so we're overfull before we know it. You might try putting your fork down between each bite. If you're fully experiencing what you're eating, you might be satisfied with one piece of candy, instead of 25.

I try to practice mindful eating and healthy eating, but I'm not a model of perfection. In the morning, I like to have a couple eggs, some whole-grain toast, or maybe some Greek yogurt, and some variation of fresh fruit. I have coffee. On the whole, I try to be cognizant and always eat breakfast and dinner together with my family.

But I also do a lot of things I shouldn't. Everyone has good days and bad days. Sometimes when I'm rushing through the airport, I grab a donut or some fast food. Part of the problem when discussing healthy eating is that people who often seem to talk the loudest are the ones who are running ultra-marathons and living on bean sprouts and snail milk. Those guys drive me crazy. Most of us aren't designed to be like that, and it presents a frustrating image and an unreachable goal. This leads people just to give up.

It's not that we shouldn't keep working toward what's optimal for us; we should, but healthy eating for each person is different. The main thing is that you keep taking small steps forward. The same holds true for exercise. Often when people start an exercise program, they dive in headfirst and then hurt themselves or get burned out. We see a lot of the weekend warrior mentality or the New Year's approach where people overestimate how much they'll be able to achieve.

Instead of starting off thinking about running the half-marathon, first, consider how fit you are and then take gradual steps toward getting more physically active based on what makes the most sense for you. You might try tai chi for a month or yoga with the goal of increasing the flexibility in your joints and back. Remember, you have to work with what's in your own personal toolkit.

It's also important to remember that being fit means different things to different people. When you feel fit, you can do all the activities you want without discomfort. Then there's cardiovascular fitness, where your heart rate slows to a healthy level, your blood pressure is well-controlled, and there are other indicators of good health that can be measured. Being able to fit into a size 2 dress or having a certain kind of body shape is not fitness.

There are markers we can look at such as blood sugar and blood pressure—those are good markers, but we're all built differently. We have to find a daily activity we like to do and find something meaningful we enjoy. This is a major-league shift. Focus on your overall health and wellness, not what you look like or how many miles you can run.

There are some really great health benefits to exercise. Several studies have shown that aerobic exercise, such as walking, bicycling, swimming, and dancing, reduce age-related brain shrinkage while improving memory and other cognitive functions. For example, a randomized controlled trial involving 120 older adults found that aerobic exercise increases the size of the anterior hippocampus in the brain, leading to improvements in spatial memory. More recent studies show that aerobic exercise increases hippocampal volume and improves memory in multiple sclerosis patients, and in older men with coronary artery disease, it correlates with an increased density of gray matter in the brain.

Exercise also strengthens your cardiovascular and respiratory systems and reduces the buildup of harmful deposits in your arteries by increasing the concentration of high-density lipoprotein—HDL or good cholesterol—in your blood. It strengthens your heart so it can pump blood more efficiently. And that reduces the risk of developing high blood pressure.

Exercise keeps bones and muscles strong by maintaining bone density, which plays several roles in preventing osteoporosis. And of course, it helps manage your weight, improving diseases and conditions associated with being overweight such as diabetes. Exercise appears to reduce your risk of certain cancers—colon, prostate, breast, uterine, and maybe others.

Exercise also helps you sleep better. Moderate exercise, at least three hours before bedtime can help you relax and sleep better at night. A good night's sleep helps maintain your physical and mental health.

Although researchers say that larger studies are needed to confirm these findings, some research shows that moderate aerobic exercise may help prevent the common cold. Those who have found that exercise does help suggest that it has a positive effect on the cells that impact your immune system.

There are psychological benefits to exercise as well. Exercise raises endorphins which gives you energy and increases serotonin which helps you sleep better. In fact, many of the things we try to accomplish with drugs, we can do with exercise and a lot more safely. Exercise also brings a sense of accomplishment; maybe you could only walk 10 minutes at a time, but now you can walk 15. That provides good motivation to help keep pushing forward.

Exercise also enhances the power of connection. Many fitness activities and sports involve other people. A researcher did an analysis of a large cross-country ski race in Minnesota. It's a solo sport, but what he found is that these extreme athletes had developed a strong community. They shared exercise tips and recipes for good food.

Exercise can also be a spiritual experience, particularly if you're doing something in nature. Some runners say that running in the woods helps them become more mindful and aware. Other people find a spiritual component when they're enjoying a day on the lake in a kayak or a canoe.

Now at this point, I'm supposed to say something like, "Check with your doctor before engaging in physical activity," but with all these benefits, maybe I should say, "Check with your doctor before not engaging in physical activity." That's where the real danger to our health lies.

A big part of what makes our modern lifestyle so unhealthy revolves around stress. We're too stressed to eat properly or to find time to exercise. Instead, we eat chips and chocolate and cookies because they're comfort food, and by golly, we need a little comfort. We lie awake at night worrying about our jobs or our finances or our kids or our parents, so we don't sleep all that well. We drink coffee and sodas for the caffeine to keep us alert enough to do our jobs. And then we're so exhausted at the end of the day that about all we can do is veg out in front of the TV. And maybe we have a drink or two—or too many—to unwind before falling exhausted, but still wired, into bed. That's what stress does to us.

It works in the other direction too. When we eat too much and sleep too little and exercise not at all, we get even more stressed. And the more we go around on that vicious cycle, the harder it is to get off. In my mind, stress is as important a factor to poor health as cigarette smoking or obesity and probably contributes to them as well and vice versa. No one can avoid stress altogether, but how you manage it is critical to your health and well-being. And there are many complementary practices that can help you do that.

We have stress responses and relaxation responses. The stress response is the fight or flight response. If a bus is about to hit you, you don't want to stop and think, "Hey, that's a 1984 Greyhound." You want to jump out of the way. It's a beautiful response because you didn't have to think about it. Your body automatically pumped up your heart rate, increased the blood flow to your muscles, while shutting off the blood flow to less vital body functions so you could jump.

But most of the stresses we face today don't require a fight or flight response. For example, if you're stuck in traffic or your spouse yells at you or the boss dumps three extra things on your desk, increasing your heart rate isn't going to help you deal with these kinds of stresses. Yet we use that same stress response over and over, day after day, and this response becomes our default pathway. It sends out adrenaline day after day, increasing our heart rate. It suppresses our immune system, and it increases inflammation, all of which lead to problems if they occur all the time for a long time.

It may sound like a contradiction, but for most of us, relaxation takes effort. You have to practice creating the relaxation response, essentially the exact opposite of what happens in the stress response. Most of us are so overwhelmed that we have to take a formal approach, such as practicing meditation or deep breathing, to see our heart rate come down, our breathing slow and our brain begin to focus on the present moment.

Sometimes you have to stop and get off the grid to realize how bad it is. When you're in that whirlwind, when your email list is 300 messages long, it's very hard to step back and realize, "Oh, I'm clenching my teeth, my shoulders are rock-hard, and my heart is racing." That's when you realize that your shoulder muscles are as tight as banjo strings, and they're not supposed to feel that way.

There's a tremendous amount of research on stress and how it impacts people's lives. From a cultural standpoint, we brag about stress. We have 14 things to do at work. We're on the cell phone while we're driving. We brag about how busy we are. That's sort of the warrior mentality.

But we know now that all those stressful situations have a cumulative effect on the body and produce a lot of negative consequences. We know that stress increases inflammation throughout your body, which creates a cascade effect that can lead to a variety of chronic diseases. For example, there's a lot of interesting data involving the heart and stress. For instance, we know that when the heart is under chronic stress, its arteries are less flexible. The heart also beats more quickly, making you more susceptible to heart rhythm disorders and chest pain. Although there's a long-standing perception that if you're a Type A personality, acute stress may increase your risk of a heart attack, stress isn't good for your heart no matter what your personality type.

Some people develop stomach problems when they're stressed. This happens because stress hormones reduce the release of stomach acid and slow stomach emptying. Stress can affect the immune system by producing the hormone cortisol which increases your susceptibility to colds and flu. We've also found that stress decreases wound healing. One study found that it took 60% longer for wounds to heal in people who were under stress than in those who weren't.

Other studies suggest that stress may worsen asthma symptoms, skin disorders, chronic pain, and depression. Children who are stressed have also been found to get sick more often. We need to start thinking of stress less as a badge of courage and more as a red flag. In my practice, I try to treat stress as aggressively as I do high cholesterol or high blood pressure.

Rest and relaxation are the best antidotes to stress, and they're as fundamental to your health as physical activity and a nutritious diet. We know we should get a good night's sleep, but somehow it always seems to end up at the bottom of the list. One of the best drivers of good sleep is how much exercise we get during the day. Twenty years ago, people were more active during the day, but now most of us stare at a computer screen for 8 hours. Because we don't have the physical and mental boost that comes from more exercise, we start feeling droopy and then we have our third cup of coffee.

Then at 8:00 or 9:00 at night, we're looking at our iPads or smartphones. A lot of us take our electronic devices to bed with us, and the artificial light from those screens suppresses melatonin, the hormone our bodies make to tell us when it's time to sleep. When combined, lack of exercise, caffeine, and electronic devices are the antithesis of what we know about good sleep habits.

If you're like many people, it's hard to keep the wheels from spinning in your head. You're thinking about what happened today and already getting prepared to fight tomorrow's battles. It can be hard to calm down, to stop the wheels from spinning and just be present in the moment. As long as the adrenaline keeps surging, you keep feeling stressed. This is where making time for rest and relaxation can help.

Rest and relaxation have a definite impact on your health. They both help you slow your heart rate, so your heart doesn't have to work as hard.

Relaxation lowers blood pressure and increases blood flow to your major muscles. Regular, deep sleep can improve immune function and reduce signs and symptoms of illness, such as headaches, nausea, diarrhea, and pain.

A good night's sleep gives you more energy and improves your concentration during the day. Believe it or not, it can also help you lose weight. When we're tired, we tend to eat more high-calorie foods to keep our energy up. When we're well rested, we don't need those calories to stay alert.

Most people need 7–8 hours of sleep a night. People who say they do fine on 5 or 6 are often doing it with lots of caffeine. Set aside adequate time for sleep and see how many of the tasks on your list you can get done in the time remaining. You may be surprised.

If you have trouble sleeping or if you just want to improve how well you sleep, some simple changes in your daily routine may help. Develop and stick to a sleep routine. Reading a book is how many people lull themselves to sleep. Some gentle tai chi may help you relax. Turn off the TV and all other electronic devices about an hour before bed.

Cut down on caffeine, especially in the hours before bedtime. Non-herbal teas, iced tea, and many soft drinks have caffeine as well as coffee and even chocolate—especially dark chocolate—has some, so look for all sources. If you're used to drinking a lot of caffeine and you cut back suddenly, you may have a headache or be unusually sleepy for a couple of days, but you'll soon feel better, and your sleep quality will improve. Avoid alcohol and nicotine before bedtime too. They both interfere with healthy sleep. If you're bothered by heartburn, don't eat a few hours before you lie down.

Avoid trying to sleep or worrying about not getting enough sleep; doing so is likely to keep you awake. And don't keep checking the clock to see how late it is. Hide your alarm clock in a drawer or turn it away from you if you find yourself looking at it too often. A surprising number of people seem to pride themselves on how little sleep they get. I'm sure you've heard a coworker bragging about getting only 4 hours of sleep the night before. Don't join that competition. Sleep is good for you; treasure it.

Although there are both prescription and nonprescription medications to help you sleep, they generally aren't recommended for long-term use. Fortunately, there are many complementary treatments for insomnia. Melatonin is a hormone produced naturally in the brain, and although melatonin supplements are widely used for jet lag, sometimes people take them to help them sleep. Melatonin is widely considered safe, but it may cause clotting problems in people taking blood thinners such as warfarin, also known as Coumadin. Also, don't take it if you're pregnant or trying to become pregnant.

The plant-based supplement valerian may help you get to sleep faster and improve sleep quality. Valerian is also used for anxiety. Research from a multi-center study found that a combination of valerian and hops may help treat insomnia. Discuss valerian with your doctor before trying it. Some people who have used high doses or used it for a long term may have increased their risk of liver damage, although it's not clear if valerian actually caused the damage.

Acupuncture and hypnosis are also commonly used to help with insomnia, although research is unclear about their value. Some people say that the smell of lavender helps put them in a peaceful frame of mind as well.

Don't ignore sleep problems that persist. People with chronic insomnia are more likely to develop psychiatric problems such as depression and anxiety disorders. Long-term sleep deprivation can also increase the severity of chronic disease such as high blood pressure and diabetes.

So whether we are sick or well, integrative medicine can help all of us achieve a healthier and more mindful way of living. Good nutrition, exercise, relaxation, and sleep are the pillars of our well-being. In the remaining lectures, we'll explore in more detail some of the ways we can use complementary and alternative approaches effectively and safely, as well as the important research that underlines use.

Lecture 3

Herbal Supplements

Dietary supplements are by far the most common form of complementary and alternative medicine, accounting for nearly 20 percent of all complementary and integrative therapy in the United States. There has been a tremendous explosion in the use of supplements since 1994, when the U.S. Congress passed the Dietary Supplement Health and Education Act, which exempts manufacturers from having to prove the efficacy and safety of their products. As you will learn in this lecture, before taking any herbal supplements, do your homework on them and involve your health-care team in the decision.

Herbal Medicine

- Herbal medicine is the practice of using plants—their roots, leaves, berries, seeds, bark, and flowers—to treat illness. Herbal supplements may come in the form of powders, pills, syrups, juices, teas, creams, or lotions. Herbal medicine has been around for a long time. As science has evolved, the healing components of many plants have been identified, extracted, and often improved to become standard drugs.

- People also turn to herbal remedies to try to prevent diseases such as Alzheimer's disease and heart disease, to manage symptoms of menopause and conditions such as fibromyalgia and osteoarthritis, and to improve their general health and well-being.

- There are marketing claims that certain herbs can cure cancer, high blood pressure, obesity, sexual problems, and depression, but there's no hard scientific evidence that any of those claims are true. Herbal supplements are best used to help prevent certain diseases, manage specific conditions or symptoms, and maintain good health—they aren't cure-alls.

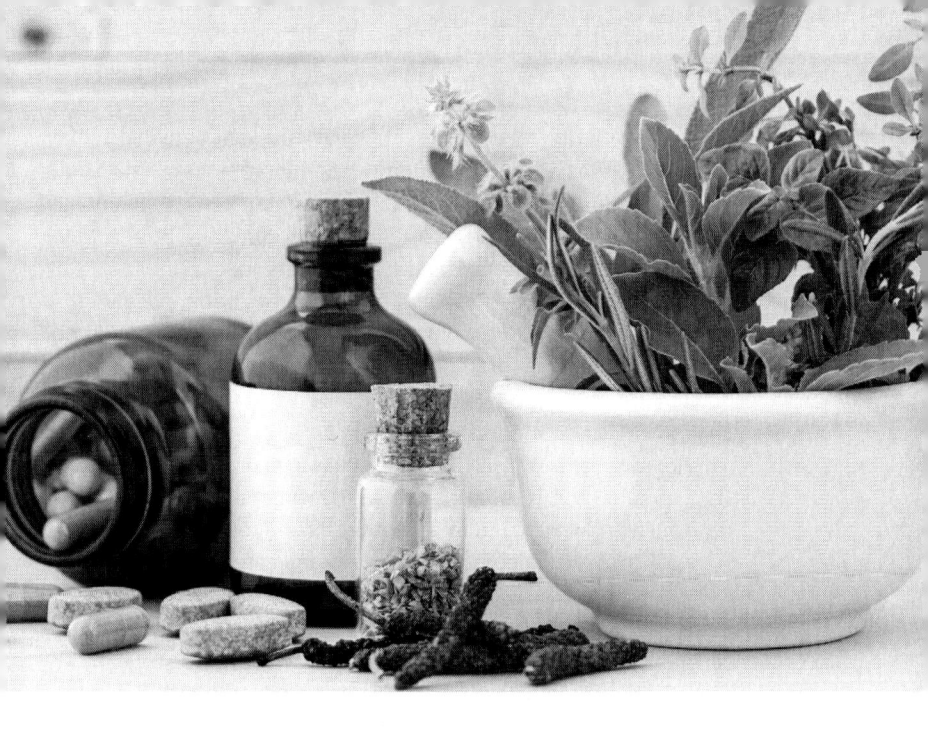

- Therefore, it's important to pay attention to the messages you read about herbs and supplements. Companies that make supplements can give you three different types of information about their products.

  1. Health claims tell you about a product's link to a disease or health condition.

  2. Nutrient claims tell you how much of a nutrient or dietary substance is in a product.

  3. Structure or function claims tell you about the intended benefits of taking the product.

- But supplements manufacturers can't just say anything they want—this is especially important when it comes to claims about what a product can do. If a supplement maker wants to say something about its product's effects, the company has to have data to back up its claims, and these claims must be followed by a statement that says, "This statement has not been evaluated by the U.S. Food and Drug Administration (FDA). This product is not intended to diagnose, treat, cure or prevent any disease."

- The federal government takes false claims about what a supplement can do very seriously. It's illegal to make claims that products can treat, prevent, or cure diseases, and the government has taken legal action against companies that promote or sell dietary products by making false statements about what they can do.

- But in the end, many consumers are still frustrated and confused by messages that are used in ads. This is when it pays to do your homework. Really look into what an advertisement claims a supplement can do and see if there's actually evidence to prove that it's true.

- Although there are some herbal remedies with good scientific evidence as to their efficacy, there are many popular herbal products without scientific evidence to back them up.

- We also know that there are risks when someone takes too many supplements—herb-herb interactions, herb-drug interactions, and so on. Supplements should not be the first thing you reach for; they should be "supplemental" to your health strategy.

- The use of complementary and alternative therapies is highest in people who have unresolved symptoms. The number one reason is back pain, followed by neck pain, joint pain or stiffness, and then arthritis. Those conditions are usually chronic, which means that you're dealing with the symptoms over a long period of time.

- Sometimes conventional drugs are very helpful for chronic conditions; other times they aren't. Or, conventional drugs may work, but they carry significant side effects. Many people with chronic conditions are interested in complementary therapies, and many are already using supplements.

Scientific Testing

- Many people are disappointed when a supplement doesn't work like the miracle drug they envisioned. Herbs and vitamins can be beneficial, but they're not the foundation of good health.

- We can test herbal therapies for efficacy and safety, just as we test prescription drugs. Many herbal therapies, however, haven't been well tested or well researched. Many of them need more rigorous scientific study.

- What constitutes a good test or good study? In general, the larger the study the better. When a study involves several hundred people or more—particularly if it lasts for several months, or even years—it gains more credibility. How the study was performed is also important. Prospective double-blind studies that have been conducted in carefully controlled, randomized settings and published in a peer-reviewed journal are the gold standard.

- Unfortunately, many herbal products haven't gone through rigorous scientific testing. The only research available are small clinical trials, poorly controlled trials, or even biased trials, where the results may be intentionally skewed to look more conclusive than they really are.

- So, in this day and age, why isn't there proper testing for herbal products? One reason is that proper testing, with good controls, is hugely expensive. This is one of the reasons for the formation of the National Center for Complementary and Integrative Health (NCCIH), a government agency under the umbrella of the National Institutes of Health.

- Many of the research studies on herbal medicines have been funded or co-funded through the NCCIH, and more testing is planned for the future. But right now, for many herbal remedies, we just don't know how effective, or even safe, they are.

Risks with Herbal Remedies

- There are also a number of other risks with herbal remedies. One is the perception that herbal products are safe because they're natural. Natural doesn't always translate into being safe—just think of tobacco or poison ivy. And any product that's strong enough to provide a potential benefit to the body can also be strong enough to cause harm.

- Another challenge has been the quality of herbs and supplements sold in the United States. Unfortunately, there are numerous examples of people being harmed by products that contained the wrong herb or that were adulterated with actual prescription drugs.

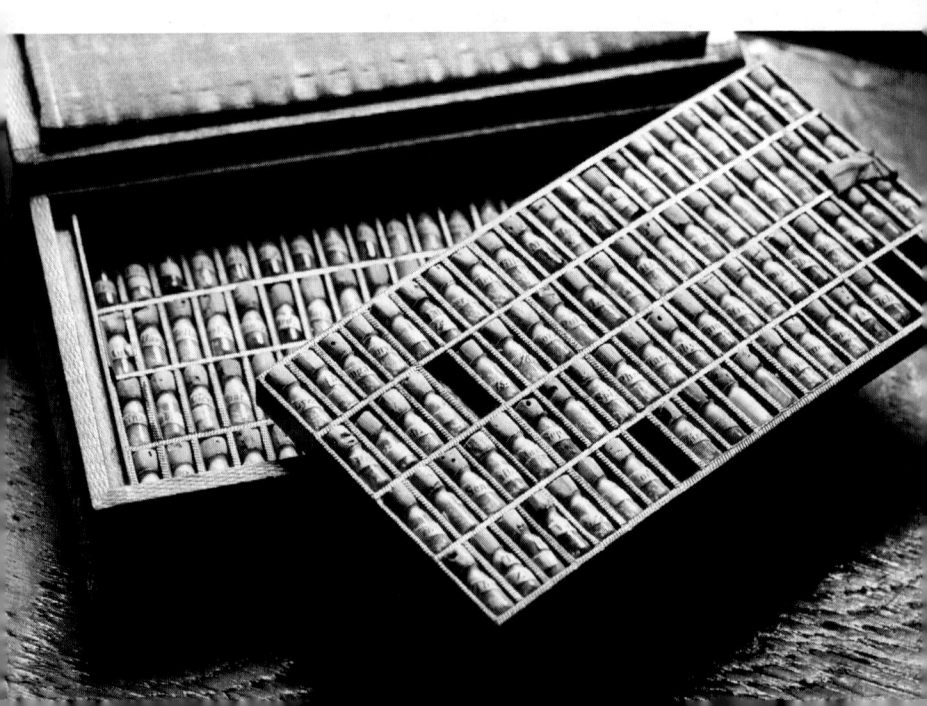

- Fortunately, thanks to some new rules called Good Manufacturing Practices, which were implemented in 2010, now all supplements sold in the United States are mandated to have in the bottle exactly what is stated on the label.

- Yet another risk is the possibility of an herbal medicine interacting in a bad way with another drug that you're taking. In a 2010 report, Mayo Clinic researchers found more than 25 herbal products that can be dangerous for heart patients on medication.

- One thing that makes this problem even more dangerous is that many people are reluctant to tell their physicians about the supplements they're taking. But it's extremely important to let your doctor know all of the things you're taking so that he or she can check for dangerous interactions with other medicines you're taking.

- Certain people should be extra careful about dietary supplements of all kinds. It's generally wise to avoid supplements if you are pregnant or breastfeeding, unless your doctor specifically approves; are having surgery; are younger than 18 or older than 65; or are already taking prescription or nonprescription medications.

- There is good information on the Internet about herbal supplements, but there's also a lot of hype and a lot of bad information. If what you read sounds too good to be true, it probably is. Make an effort to seek out a reliable, authoritative source. When you're looking for information about herbal supplements on the Internet, remember the three Ds.

    1. Date: Check the creation or update date on the website. If you don't see a date, don't assume that the information is recent. Older material may be outdated and not include recent findings.

    2. Documentation: Check the sources. Are qualified health professionals creating and reviewing the information? Is

advertising clearly identified? Look for the logo from the Health on the Net Foundation, which means that the information follows their principles for reliability and credibility.

3. Double-check: Visit several health sites and compare the information they offer. If you can't find any supporting evidence to back up the claims of an alternative product, be skeptical.

- Before you follow any advice you find on the Internet, check with your doctor for guidance.

- Mayo Clinic evaluates many herbal supplements and offers information online at mayoclinic.org/drugs-supplements, and the NCCIH website has a feature called "Herbs at a Glance," which gives you up-to-date, unbiased information, as well as links to peer-reviewed scientific articles on the research of various herbs.

- When you've done your research and checked with your doctor, the next step is to head to a pharmacy or store that sells herbal products. But how do you choose the right brand?

    o Look for standardized supplements. The U.S. Pharmacopeial Convention's (USP) dietary supplement verification seal on the label indicates that the product has met certain manufacturing standards. Other groups that certify supplements include ConsumerLab.com and NSF International.

    o Look for a large, recognizable manufacturer.

    o Be cautious about supplements made outside the United States.

- Bodybuilding and weight loss are two big reasons people use herbal supplements—and they're two types of supplements that have caused a lot of problems. Some companies add other ingredients to these supplements that aren't safe, including stimulants. Keep in mind that any product that's strong enough to make you lose weight quickly is going to affect other parts of your body, such as your heart.

- Before you buy a supplement, in addition to doing your research, also consider the cost. Spending $45 a week on something you're not even sure will work might not be the answer you're looking for. It's all about being a well-informed and wise consumer.

Dangerous Herbal Products

- There are certain herbal products that can be very dangerous. For example, kava is a member of the pepper family whose root and underground stem are used in various forms to treat anxiety, insomnia, and menopausal symptoms. But the FDA has issued a warning that using kava supplements can cause severe liver damage, including hepatitis and liver failure, possibly leading to death. Kava may also interact unfavorably with several drugs.

- Another herbal supplement to beware of is ephedra, whose main active ingredient, ephedrine, is known to stimulate the nervous system and heart. It has been used as an ingredient in dietary supplements designed to help people lose weight, boost their energy, and improve their athletic performance. However, between 1995 and 1997, the FDA received more than 900 reports of possible ephedra toxicity. In 2004, the FDA banned the sale of dietary supplements containing ephedra in the United States.

- Yohimbe, a supplement that promises sexual potency and pleasure, lowers blood pressure and increases blood flow to the genitals. It's used to treat sexual dysfunction. Yohimbe can cause severe side effects, including high blood pressure, a racing heartbeat, kidney failure, headache, anxiety, dizziness, nausea, vomiting, tremors, and sleeplessness. The herb can be very dangerous if you take too much of it or take it over a long period of time.

Suggested Reading

Barton, et al, "Pilot Study of Panax Quinquefolius (American Ginseng) to Improve Cancer-Related Fatigue."

Buenz, et al, "Bioprospecting Rumphius's Ambonese Herbal."

ConsumerLab.com, "How to Read a ConsumerLab.com Approved Quality Product Seal."

Edakkanambeth, et al, "Over-the-Counter Enzyme Supplements."

Hurt, et al, "L-Arginine for the Treatment of Centrally Obese Subjects."

Mayo Clinic, "Drugs and Supplements."

McGarey, *Physician within You.*

National Center for Complementary and Integrative Health, "Herbs at a Glance."

NSF International, "What Is NSF Certification?"

Sood, et al, "A Randomized Clinical Trial of St. John's Wort for Smoking Cessation."

Thompson, et al, "Dietary Supplement S-Adenosyl-L-Methionine (AdoMet) Effects on Plasma Homocysteine Levels in Healthy Human Subjects."

United States Pharmacopeia, "USP Verification Services."

Lecture 3 Transcript

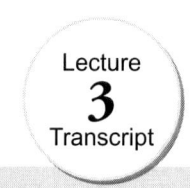

Herbal Supplements

In the United States, dietary supplements—herbs, vitamins, even a few hormones—are a $30-billion a year business. You could run a small country on that kind of money. Dietary supplements are by far the most common form of complementary and alternative medicine, accounting for nearly 20% of all complementary and integrative therapy in the United States. More than 30% of adults in the United States use herbs and other supplements. Worldwide, that number is closer to 80%.

There's been a tremendous explosion in the use of supplements since 1994 when the United States Congress passed the Dietary Supplement Health and Education Act. The FDA originally proposed enhanced oversight of supplement manufacturers in response to some serious adverse effects traced back to specific herbs and supplements. But the industry pushed back in a big way, and eventually, Congress passed this law, which basically created the category of dietary supplements, and in the end, resulted in a lot less oversight power than what the FDA had originally proposed.

There are two critical parts of the dietary supplement act that deserve special attention. First, manufacturers are exempted from having to prove efficacy. That means they are not required to do formal research to prove that their product does what they claim. Second, manufacturers don't have to prove the safety of their products. They're expected to have some historical usage data to support its safety, but again, there's no requirement for specific testing to ensure a product is safe.

With these exemptions in place, the market really blossomed. Consumers started to get inundated. Information about supplements was all over the Internet. At the same time, there was a growing dissatisfaction with the current state of medicine in the United States. Patients and consumers wanted to be more engaged in their care, and the boom in supplement sales was partly due to that search for greater health care autonomy.

This isn't meant to suggest that the Food and Drug Administration isn't regulating the supplement market. The FDA does a lot to make sure the products we buy are safe and of high quality. But there's no denying that the rules Congress passed do limit the FDA in many ways. This means that as consumers, we still have work to do before we add dietary supplements to our daily health care regimen.

So, let's take a closer look and see if the $30 billion a year we put toward dietary supplements is being well spent. Let's start with herbal supplements. What's herbal medicine all about, anyway? Herbal medicine is the practice of using plants—their roots, leaves, berries, seeds, bark, and flowers—to treat illness. Herbal supplements may come in the form of powders, pills, syrups, juices, teas, creams, or lotions.

Herbal medicine has been around for a long time. As science has evolved, the healing components of many plants have been identified, extracted, and often improved to become standard drugs.

Some good examples of standard Western medicines derived from plants are: digitalis, which comes from foxglove leaves and is used to treat congestive heart failure; aspirin made from willow bark, which is taken for pain and fever; quinine from the bark of the cinchona tree, which is used to treat malaria; the powerful pain relievers morphine and codeine, which come from the opium poppy seed

People also turn to herbal remedies to try to prevent diseases such as Alzheimer's and heart disease, to manage symptoms of menopause and conditions such as fibromyalgia and osteoarthritis, and to improve their general health and well-being.

There are marketing claims that certain herbs can cure cancer, high blood pressure, obesity, sexual problems, depression, and ingrown toenails, but there's no hard scientific evidence that any of those claims are true. In fact, the more wonderful the claim, the more likely it isn't true. Herbal supplements are best used to help prevent certain diseases, manage specific conditions or symptoms, and maintain good health. They aren't cure-alls.

With that said, it's important to pay attention to the messages you read or hear about herbs and supplements. Companies that make supplements can give you three different types of information about their products. Health claims tell you about a product's link to a disease or health condition. Nutrient claims tell you how much of a nutrient or dietary substance is in a product. Structure or function claims tell you about the intended benefits of taking the product. But supplement manufacturers can't just say anything they want. This is especially important when it comes to claims about what a product can do. If a supplement maker wants to say something about its product's effects, the company has to have data to back up its claims, and these claims must be followed by a statement that says, "This statement has not been evaluated by the U.S. Food and Drug Administration—FDA. This product is not intended to diagnose, treat, cure, or prevent any disease."

The federal government takes false claims about what a supplement can do very seriously. It's illegal to make claims that products can treat, prevent, or cure diseases, and government has taken legal action against companies that promote or sell products by making false statements about what they can do. But in the end, a lot of consumers are still frustrated and confused. Although an advertisement can't say that a supplement will reduce urinary frequency—that would be a medical claim—it can state that the supplement can be used to promote prostate health—a structure or function claim. In the end, messages that are used in ads often just confuse and sometimes deceive consumers. This is when it pays to do your homework. Really look into what an advertisement claims a supplement can do and see if there's actually evidence out there to prove that it's true.

At Mayo Clinic, many of my patients use supplements, but they use them in different ways. There are some people who come in with a shopping bag full of bottles and teas—maybe 40 or 50 different supplements they take every day. These are folks who hear a few tidbits about the latest super juice or breakthrough vitamin and rush to add it to their regimen.

You may be asking yourself, "How does anybody end up with 40 or 50 different supplements?" It's easier than you think. Your pharmacist may recommend psyllium for constipation; you might read about acai berry juice for weight loss in a magazine; perhaps you watch a talk show guest touting Echinacea for cold prevention; you see a Facebook post from a friend of a friend with a glowing endorsement of ginkgo as a brain booster, and before you know it, you're spending upwards of $100 a month on herbal supplements that you may or may not need, and that might or might not work. How do we know if any of this is good for us?

Unfortunately, in many cases, we don't know, and what we do know should probably give us pause. Although there are some herbal remedies with good scientific evidence as to their efficacy—ones that I use in my own practice, which I'll talk more about later—there are many popular herbal products without scientific evidence to back them up. They haven't been found to work any better than a placebo. That means they probably don't work, and we should be looking for other, more evidence-based places to invest our wellness dollars.

We also know that there are risks when someone takes that many supplements—herb-herb interactions, herb-drug interactions and so forth. But criticizing the person—shaming him or her—is rarely helpful. Often times, these individuals are very interested in their health, and they're trying to be proactive. So I try to start from there. I tell them that I'm glad they're interested in improving their health, but that I want them to begin by looking at their foundation. I bring up NESS. Remember? The acronym we discussed at the very beginning of this course: Nutrition, Exercise, Stress Management and Support. Once people understand that this is the foundational approach for lifelong health and wellness, we can usually shift focus away from supplements as the first thing they reach for and help them to see supplements as what they really are—supplemental to their health strategy.

After discussing the importance of a good health foundation approach, I then look at each supplement the person is taking and see where the redundancies might be. For example, maybe the person is getting Vitamin A from several different sources to the point of getting into dangerous territory.

It's important to respect a person's enthusiasm for achieving good health, but it's also important to let him or her know about the science behind the supplements they're taking so they can take a rational approach.

Then there are the people who are struggling with chronic symptoms. We know that the use of complementary and alternative therapies are highest in people who have unresolved symptoms. The number one reason is back pain, followed by neck pain, joint pain or stiffness, and then arthritis. Those conditions are usually chronic, which means that you're dealing with the symptoms over a long period of time. Sometimes conventional drugs are very helpful for chronic conditions; other times they aren't. Or conventional drugs may work, but they carry significant side effects. Many of the people I see with chronic conditions are very interested in complementary therapies, and many are already using supplements.

So individuals with arthritis are a good example. Many have tried acetaminophen but have found it isn't strong enough. Others are getting good control of their pain with NSAIDs than anti-inflammatory drugs but then they run into blood pressure or kidney problems. They've tried to lose weight, they've gone to physical therapy, but their back or their knees still hurt.

These individuals often are eager to try something new and are willing to experiment with SAMe or glucosamine and see what kind of results they get. I think this is a great opportunity for a doctor and patient to work together as partners to explore these nonprescription options, looking to see what may work and how to incorporate supplements into an overall health strategy while making sure to steer clear of side effects or adverse effects.

A lot of people are disappointed when a supplement doesn't work like the miracle drug they envisioned. Miracles are rare. If you take a garlic supplement for your heart, but you don't change your exercise or eating habits, the supplement isn't going to help you much. Herbs and vitamins can be beneficial, but they're not the foundation of good health.

Some people also say you have to believe in herbal therapy for it to work. This isn't true; we can test herbal therapies for efficacy and safety just as we test prescription drugs. Many herbal therapies, however, haven't been well tested or well researched. Many of them need more rigorous scientific study. You may be wondering, what constitutes a good study or a good test?

In general, the larger the study, the better. When a study involves several hundred people or more—particularly if it lasts over several months or even years—it gains more credibility. How the study was performed is also important. Prospective, double-blind studies that have been conducted in carefully controlled, randomized settings and published in a peer-reviewed journal are really the gold standard.

When you're evaluating a scientific study for an herbal supplement, look for clinical studies that involve human beings, not animals. They're usually preceded by studies that demonstrate safety and effectiveness when used in animals. Mice and men have many genes in common, but a man is still not a mouse.

In what's called a controlled trial, participants are usually divided into two groups. The first group receives the treatment being studied. The second is a control group. People in this group receive the standard treatment, no treatment, or an inactive substance called a placebo. What researchers have discovered is that people who think they're getting the real medicine when it's really just a placebo or a sugar pill, sometimes get better. This remarkable and quite real benefit is called the placebo effect, and it's a good example of how our minds and beliefs can affect our bodies.

We gather evidence about a dietary supplement the same way we gather evidence about prescription drugs—by conducting fair tests. Researchers study whether the supplement causes an improvement beyond the improvement caused by the placebo effect alone. Of course, improvement due to the placebo effect is still improvement, and that's always welcome. But it's important to remember that for many health conditions, there are treatments that work better than placebo treatments. If you choose a treatment that provides only a placebo effect, you may miss out on the benefits that a more effective treatment could provide.

To be effective, a controlled trial also needs to be randomized. That means that participants are assigned to the treatment and control groups on a random basis. This helps ensure that all the groups will be similar. In double-blind studies, neither the researchers nor the participants know who is receiving the active treatment or who is receiving the placebo. Also, peer-reviewed journals only publish articles that have been reviewed by an independent panel of experts. The peer review is usually anonymous, and the reviewers usually aren't paid. They expect that when they have research to submit, others will do the same for them.

Finally, ask yourself if the research applies to you. Here's an example. Mayo Clinic has conducted two studies to see if ginseng helps fatigue in people who've had cancer. We worked with a specific grower in Wisconsin so we could control how this particular ginseng was harvested and processed it in a uniform manner, so we knew that each capsule contained a specific amount of the active ingredients of ginseng. In this case, studies showed that ginseng helped those in the study group feel less fatigued.

But that doesn't necessarily mean it'll have the same effect for you. If you're not buying the same kind of ginseng that was in the study, or you're not a cancer survivor, you might not see the same results. So when you're looking at research, look not only for good-quality studies but also studies that you can relate to based on your goals for taking a supplement in the first place.

Unfortunately, many herbal products haven't gone through rigorous scientific testing. The only research available are small clinical trials, poorly controlled trials, or even biased trials, where the results may be intentionally skewed to look more conclusive than they really are. So, in this day and age, why isn't there proper testing for herbal products?

One reason is that proper testing, with good controls, is hugely expensive. Pharmaceutical companies are willing to test prescription drugs because they stand to make a great deal of money out of a successful drug that they can patent. But you can't patent garlic, or rose hips, or ginkgo leaves, or any plant for that matter. So anybody can make and sell herbal remedies. Plus, who's going to pay all that money to have the products properly tested and possibly discredited?

This was one of the reasons for the formation of the National Center for Complementary and Integrative Health, or NCCIH, a government agency under the umbrella of the National Institutes of Health. Their mission is "to define, through rigorous scientific investigation, the usefulness, and safety of complementary and integrative health interventions and their roles in improving health and health care."

Many of the research studies on herbal medicines have been funded or co-funded through the NCCIH, and more testing is planned for the future. But right now, for a lot of herbal remedies, we just don't know how effective or even how safe they are.

There are a number of other risks with herbal remedies too. One is the perception that herbal products are safe because they're natural. As we've talked about before, natural doesn't always translate into being safe—just think of tobacco, strychnine, or poison ivy. And of course, any product that's strong enough to provide a potential benefit to the body can also be strong enough to cause harm.

Another challenge has been quality of herbs and supplements sold in the United States. The Dietary Supplement Health and Education Act of 1994 didn't really give the Food and Drug Administration sufficient authority or resources to ensure the quality of dietary supplements sold in the U.S. Unfortunately, there are numerous examples of people being harmed by products that contained the wrong herb or that were adulterated with actual prescription medications. Many herbal remedies produced in China, for example, have been found to contain toxic amounts of heavy metals such as arsenic, lead, and mercury. And even when people aren't harmed, paying a hefty price for a product that doesn't contain any of the herb you think you're buying is a pretty poor investment.

Fortunately, thanks to some new rules called GMPs—Good Manufacturing Practices—which were implemented in 2010, now all supplements sold in the United States are mandated to have in the bottle exactly what is stated on the label. There are probably still some bad actors out there—mostly fly-by-night internet setups—but finding good-quality products is becoming easier. This, at least, helps remove one barrier to the safe use of herbs and supplements.

Yet another risk is the possibility of an herbal medication interacting in a bad way with another drug that you're taking. For example, we know that St. John's wort can produce dangerous reactions with certain prescription drugs. Patients have experienced heart transplant rejection when they combined St. John's wort with their anti-rejection medications.

In a 2010 report, Mayo Clinic researchers found more than 25 herbal products that can be dangerous for heart patients on medication. Herbal remedies such as ginseng, ginkgo, garlic, black cohosh, St. John's wort, hawthorn, saw palmetto, and Echinacea can dilute, intensify, or exacerbate the side effects of prescription heart drugs such as blood thinners and cholesterol-lowering statins. Some supplements may also increase heart rate and blood pressure, causing potential complications in heart patients.

One thing that makes this problem even more dangerous is that many people are reluctant to tell their physicians about the supplements they're taking. They may think that since herbs are natural, it's not a big deal. Or they may be afraid that the doctor will lecture them for using herbal medicines at all. And it's true that not all doctors are accepting or even knowledgeable about herbal treatments. But let me tell you, it's really, really important to let your doctor know all the things you're taking so he or she can check for dangerous interactions with other medications you're taking. It could literally save your life.

There are some people who should be extra careful about dietary supplements of all kinds. It's generally wise to avoid supplements if you're pregnant or breastfeeding unless your doctor specifically approves. Medication that may be safe for you as an adult may be harmful to your baby or to your breastfeeding infant. If you're having surgery; some herbal supplements can decrease the effectiveness of anesthesia or cause dangerous complications such as bleeding or high blood pressure. Tell your doctor about any herbs you're taking or considering as soon as you know you need surgery.

You'll need to take extra precaution if you're younger than 18 or older than 65. Older adults may metabolize medications differently, and few supplements have been studied on children or have established safe doses for children. It's especially important to talk to your doctor first if you're already taking prescription or nonprescription medications. Some herbs can cause serious side effects when mixed with other drugs, such as aspirin.

There is good information on the Internet about herbal supplements, but there's also a lot of hype and a lot of bad information. If what you read sounds too good to be true, it probably is. Make an effort to seek out a reliable, authoritative source. When you're looking for information about herbal supplements on the internet, remember the Three Ds.

Date: check out the creation or update date on the website. If you don't see a date, don't assume the information is recent. Older material may be outdated and not include recent findings.

Documentation: check the sources. Are qualified health professionals creating and reviewing the information? Academic centers are required to release any conflicts of interests the authors may have such as serving on pharmaceutical boards or accepting grant money from certain companies, but private groups are not. Is advertising clearly identified? Look for the logo from the Health on the Net Foundation, which means that it follows the HON principles for reliability and credibility of information.

Double-check: visit several health sites and compare the information they offer. If you can't find any supporting evidence to back up the claims of an alternative product, be skeptical.

And before you follow any advice you find on the internet, check with your doctor for guidance. Gather the information you've found, and ask, "Given what you know about my health, do you think this would be helpful? Does it interact with any of the medications I'm taking?" These questions are critical to making sure that what you're taking makes good sense for you and that it's safe for you to take.

Mayo Clinic evaluates many herbal supplements and offers information online at mayoclinic.org/drugs-supplements, and the NCCIH website has a feature called Herbs at a Glance. It gives you up-to-date, unbiased information, as well as links to peer-reviewed scientific articles on the research of various herbs.

When you've done your research and checked with your doctor, next up is to head to a pharmacy or store that sells herbal products. There you may find 15 kinds of ginkgo supplements and more ginseng than you ever imagined. How do you choose the right brand?

Look for standardized supplements. The U.S. Pharmacopeia's USP dietary supplement verification seal on the label indicates that the product has met certain manufacturing standards. Other groups that certify supplements include ConsumerLab.com and NSF International. Although each group takes a slightly different approach, the goal of each is to certify the product meets a certain standard.

Also, look for a large, recognizable manufacturer. While this isn't a guarantee that the product contains exactly what it says it does, chances are better that a well-known company with a good reputation will make the effort to produce a quality product. Be cautious about supplements made outside the United States. Many European herbs and other dietary supplements are highly regulated and standardized. But toxic ingredients and prescription drugs have been found in some supplements manufactured in other countries.

Bodybuilding and weight loss are two big reasons people use herbal supplements, and they're two types of supplements that have caused a lot of problems. Some companies add other ingredients to these supplements that aren't safe, including stimulants. The main thing to keep in mind with these supplements is this: Any product that's strong enough to make you lose weight quickly is going to affect other parts of your body, such as your heart.

Before you buy a supplement, in addition to doing your research, also consider the cost. Spending $45 a week on something you're not even sure will work might not be the answer you're looking for. It's all about being a well-informed and wise consumer. In the next lecture, I'm going to discuss a number of popular supplements. But there are certain herbal products that can be very dangerous, and I want to address these first.

Kava is a member of the pepper family whose root and underground stem, called the rhizome, are used in various forms to treat anxiety, insomnia, and menopausal symptoms. Scientific studies provide some evidence that kava may help manage anxiety, but the FDA has issued a warning that using kava supplements can cause severe liver damage, including hepatitis and liver failure, possibly leading to death. Kava may also interact unfavorably with several other drugs, including drugs used to treat Parkinson's disease.

Another herbal supplement to be aware of is ephedra, whose main active ingredient, ephedrine, is known to stimulate the nervous system and heart. It has been used as an ingredient in dietary supplements designed to help people lose weight, boost their energy, and improve their athletic performance. These marketing claims made ephedra very attractive to a wide range of people, but the science doesn't support the hype.

Between 1995 and 1997, the FDA received more than 900 reports of possible ephedra toxicity. Serious adverse events such as stroke, heart attack, and sudden death were reported in 37 cases. In 2001, a Minnesota Vikings lineman died after collapsing during one of the team's summer workouts, and in 2003, Baltimore Orioles pitcher Steve Bechler died during spring training. Products containing ephedra were linked to both deaths.

In 2004, the FDA banned the sale of dietary supplements containing ephedra in the United States. But it's important to note that this ban doesn't apply to traditional Chinese herbal remedies or to products like herbal teas regulated as conventional foods.

Bitter orange is a tree whose oil is used in foods, cosmetics, and aromatherapy products. After ephedra was banned, many herbal weight-loss products began using concentrated extracts of bitter orange peel instead of ephedra. But it's important to note that bitter orange contains the chemical synephrine, which is similar to the main chemical in ephedra.

Presently, there's not a lot of evidence that bitter orange is any safer than ephedra, or that taking it will result in permanent weight loss.

And then there's yohimbe. If there's a holy grail of herbal supplements, a product that people are interested in even more than one that touts dramatic weight loss, it's a supplement that promises sexual potency and pleasure. And that's what's claimed for yohimbe. The bark of the yohimbe tree contains a chemical called yohimbine. As a dietary supplement, the dried bark of the yohimbe tree is made into tea and taken by mouth. An extract of the bark is also put into capsules and tablets.

Yohimbine lowers blood pressure and increases blood flow to the genitals. Traditionally, it's been used in Africa to increase sexual desire. Currently, it's used to treat sexual dysfunction, including erectile dysfunction in men. A drug form of yohimbine called yohimbine hydrochloride has been studied for erectile dysfunction and is considered safe if taken under a doctor's supervision.

Yohimbe can cause severe side effects, including high blood pressure, a racing heartbeat, kidney failure, headache, anxiety, dizziness, nausea, vomiting, tremors, and sleeplessness. The herb can be very dangerous if you take too much of it or take it over a long period of time. Finally, it's important to know that the amount of yohimbine in dietary supplements varies widely, and some products contain very little of the herb.

We've focused on just a few herbs that we know can and have caused serious harm to many people. But I think we should be careful not to oversimplify and call some herbs bad and others good. Even a safe herb like chamomile can cause serious harm to somebody with a severe allergy to members of the Asteraceae family. And a potentially dangerous herb, such as kava, can be used effectively if it's overseen by a skilled clinician. The take-home message here is to treat all herbs and supplements with respect, do your homework, and always involve your health-care team before deciding whether or not a particular herb is right for you.

In the next lecture, we'll take a closer look at the way some popular supplements are used to treat patients with conditions commonly encountered in integrative medicine practice.

Lecture 4

Supplements in Practice

As with almost all of the therapies discussed in this course, supplements are rarely a substitute for conventional medical treatment, and they're almost never a standalone solution. First, build your NESS foundation (nutrition, exercise, stress management, and social support). Then, if you still have a persisting symptom or problem, talk to your health-care team if you're considering adding a supplement in a targeted and evidence-based fashion, and take an active role in evaluating and reevaluating your treatment as new medications and treatments become available. In this lecture, you will learn how some popular supplements are used to treat patients with conditions commonly encountered in integrative medicine practice.

Supplements for Arthritis

- Some patients are interested in trying glucosamine for arthritis pain. Many people are troubled by knee pain, particularly athletes. Because the cartilage inside our knees doesn't have a great blood supply, it often doesn't heal well after injury. Glucosamine may provide some relief.

- Glucosamine is one the most widely used dietary supplements. Our bodies naturally make glucosamine, which is an amino sugar. Glucosamine supplements sold in stores are typically made from the skeletons of shellfish, and there are several forms. The form best suited for cartilage repair appears to be glucosamine sulfate.

- Study results on glucosamine for cartilage repair have varied, but several studies show that glucosamine sulfate is helpful in treating osteoarthritis. People with osteoarthritis use supplements such as glucosamine in hopes that the supplements can improve their symptoms and reduce their need for pain-relieving medications such as nonsteroidal anti-inflammatory drugs (NSAIDs), which can be more expensive and may cause serious side effects.

- Glucosamine is often taken together with chondroitin, which also comes from cartilage, usually cow and shark cartilage. It's not clear if combining the two compounds is more effective than taking them alone.

- Studies looking at both glucosamine and chondroitin are mixed. Glucosamine and chondroitin are generally safe and may offer some relief to some people with osteoarthritis—at least some studies seem to suggest this. Along with NESS (nutrition, exercise, stress management, and social support) as the foundation, patients can try glucosamine and chondroitin for maybe three to four months before they decide whether it's helpful. Those who don't see any improvement after four months can explore other options.

- As with other types of supplements, a major issue is product quality. There's a lot of variability among glucosamine-plus-chondroitin supplements. In the past, some products contained no chondroitin despite label claims, while others contained more chondroitin than the label showed. And price isn't always a guarantee of quality. But with the current Good Manufacturing Rules now in place, finding quality supplements is getting easier.

- Another supplement that may be useful in treating arthritis is SAMe (S-adenosyl-L-methionine), a naturally occurring chemical in the human body that helps produce and regulate hormones. A synthetic version of SAMe has become a popular dietary supplement in the United States, used for arthritis, depression, and liver disease.

- SAMe has been studied extensively in the treatment of osteoarthritis. Multiple trials indicate that it can relieve pain from arthritis as effectively as NSAIDs, but with fewer side effects. However, it may take up to 30 days to get significant relief.

- Clinical trials have suggested that SAMe can also improve symptoms of fibromyalgia, which can cause chronic pain as well as depressive symptoms. SAMe isn't approved by the FDA to treat depression in the United States, but it's used in Europe as a prescription drug to treat depression. SAMe may be helpful, but more research is needed.

- SAMe can interact with drugs or supplements to affect blood pressure, blood glucose, or the risk of bleeding, so be sure your doctor is aware of everything you're taking.

- If the supplement you want to take is generally safe for your situation, you can try it for a month or two and see if you notice any improvement in symptoms. If you're not noticing a difference, stop taking it.

Supplements for the Aging Body

- Hormone therapy, in which the hormone estrogen is taken alone or combined with hormone progesterone, is used to treat symptoms of menopause. Hormone therapy may be a good choice for certain women to treat hot flashes and sleep difficulties, depending on their risk factors. But hormone therapy needs to be individualized.

- Bioidentical hormones are also used to treat symptoms of menopause. Bioidentical basically means that the hormones in the product are chemically the same as the ones in your body. However, the hormones in the bioidentical medications might not be any different than those in traditional hormone therapy.

- Because many bioidentical hormones are marketed as "natural," people think they're safer, but they aren't. And there isn't any evidence that they're more effective. "Natural" only means the hormones come from plant or animal sources—they're not synthesized in a lab. However, many of them still need to be commercially processed to become bioidentical.

- Some people view bioidentical hormones as almost magical. But they carry the same risks as hormone therapy, so you should talk with your doctor before using them. For women with severe hot flashes that interfere with their quality of life, hormone therapy many be prescribed for a short period—maybe three to five years, and possibly longer if your doctor thinks that prolonged use would be safe.

- Black cohosh, a member of the buttercup family, is a plant that was used in Native American medicine and was a home remedy for rheumatism and arthritis in 19th-century America. In recent years, black cohosh has become popular for treating hot flashes, night sweats, vaginal dryness, and other symptoms of menopause. Black cohosh has also been used for menstrual irregularities and premenstrual syndrome, and to induce labor.

- A meta-analysis of clinical trials for relief of menopausal symptoms found that black cohosh, whether used alone or with other botanicals, failed to relieve hot flashes and night sweats in postmenopausal women or those approaching menopause.

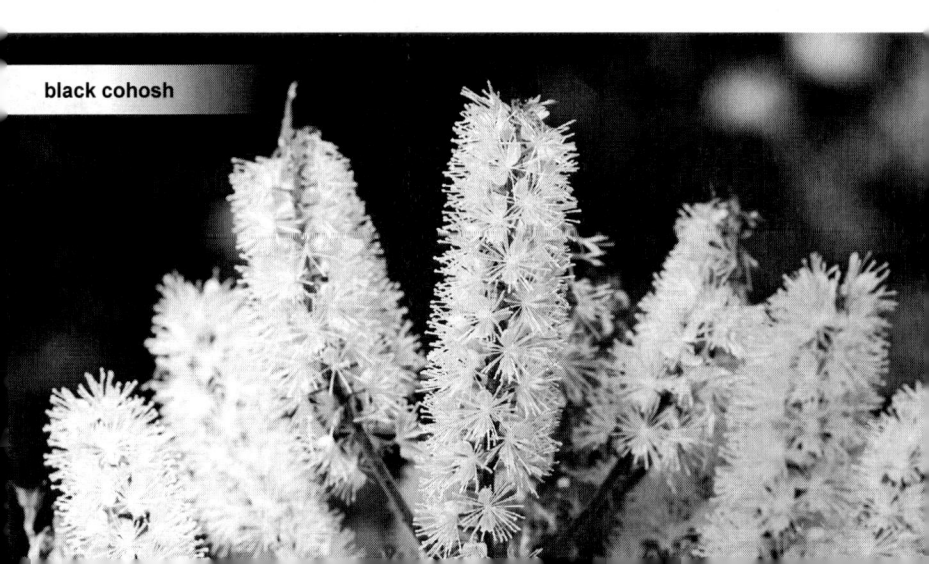

black cohosh

- For the most part, clinical trials of black cohosh to treat menopausal symptoms haven't found that the herb causes serious side effects, but some people taking black cohosh have experienced stomach discomfort, headache, or rash. Scientists are also concerned about how the herb may affect the liver.

- If you take birth control pills, hormone replacement therapy, sedatives, or blood pressure medicine, don't take black cohosh without your doctor's approval. Because hot flashes can be a difficult symptom to treat, a patient might do a trial of black cohosh, especially if she hasn't had success with conventional approaches.

- Soy is another plant that has been traditionally used to treat menopausal symptoms—as well as osteoporosis, memory problems, high blood pressure, high cholesterol levels, breast cancer, and prostate cancer. As a dietary supplement, soy is available in tablets and capsules that may contain isoflavones or phytoestrogens, soy protein, or both.

- Some studies suggest that soy isoflavone supplements may reduce hot flashes in women after menopause, but the results have been inconsistent. There's not enough scientific evidence to know if soy supplements are effective for any other health uses.

- In general, eating soy foods seems safe and may be beneficial. Taking high doses of soy supplements, on the other hand, doesn't seem to have a lot of proven benefits and may lead to some risks.

- For men, saw palmetto has been used as an alternative treatment for the urinary symptoms associated with an enlarged prostate, also called benign prostatic hyperplasia (BPH). It's also taken for chronic pelvic pain, bladder disorders, decreased sex drive, hair loss, hormone imbalances, and prostate cancer.

- BPH is such a vexing problem for many men as they age, and many conventional medicines to treat it are expensive or can have side effects. Patients can try saw palmetto to see if they get any positive results.

- Keeping a good record of your response to a supplement can really help you determine which one may be right for you.

Supplements for Heart Disease

- When it comes to preventing heart disease, it's not possible to overstate the importance of the four principles of NESS—nutrition, exercise, stress management, and social support—as an overall strategy for optimizing health and wellness.

- When we think about the sequelae of heart disease—the negative aftereffects—one of the more challenging for many patients is something called congestive heart failure, which means that the heart muscle is no longer pumping as effectively as it once did. Many patients face heart failure after having heart damage from a heart attack.

- Conventional medicine has a number of treatments (such as beta blockers and ACE inhibitors) that have been shown to reduce the risk of further heart disease and help alleviate the symptoms of heart failure. In some cases, they may even help to remodel the heart muscle back into a nearly normal function.

- For heart failure, two supplements are at the top of Natural Medicines Comprehensive Database (which is compiled by pharmacists and medical doctors): coenzyme Q10 and fish oil.

- Coenzyme Q10 is an antioxidant made by your body and used by cells throughout your body for their basic functions. It helps your body convert food into energy. Coenzyme Q10 has been shown to reduce mortality by nearly half in certain patients with moderate to severe heart failure.

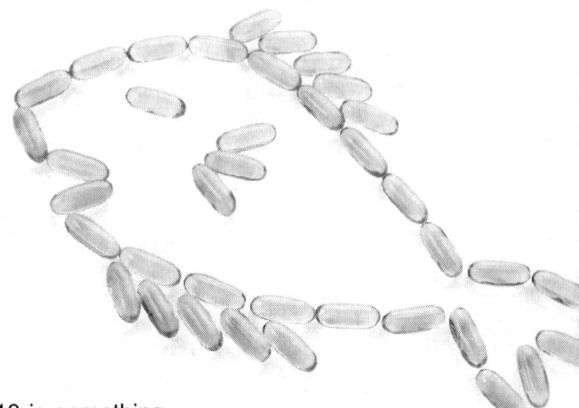

- Coenzyme Q10 is something to talk about with your health-care team if you're dealing with congestive heart failure. It's important to note to that in most of the studies on coenzyme Q10, it was used as an adjunct—which means that it was used after the conventional therapy had already been in place—so we should consider coenzyme Q10 as part of an overall strategy, not as a substitute for conventional therapy.

- Another supplement that has shown in treating congestive heart failure is fish oil, which is one of the most widely used dietary supplements in the United States.

- A meta-analysis conducted by Dr. W. Xin and colleagues in Beijing concluded that using fish oil supplements in patients with congestive heart failure resulted in a number of improvements in the overall function of the heart.

- Keep in mind that high doses of fish oil can be harmful. Too much fish oil can increase your risk of bleeding, cause higher levels of low-density lipoprotein (LDL, or "bad") cholesterol, and cause problems controlling your blood sugar.

- Simply eating more fish is part of an overall healthy nutrition strategy, but there are ongoing concerns about fish and especially the accumulation of toxic chemicals, such as mercury, that make eating fish every day at least somewhat problematic.

- Hawthorn berries have been around for a long time with a rather long history of efficacy for treating congestive heart failure. In patients who don't have access to the best conventional medical management of congestive heart failure, hawthorn probably does have something to offer. But for people who are receiving the best conventional treatments available, it seems like hawthorn probably falls by the wayside.

- Patients who have congestive heart failure and are interested in dietary supplements can explore possibly using coenzyme Q10 and fish oil. But the evidence on hawthorn is somewhat conflicting.

Suggested Reading

Clegg, et al, "Glucosamine, Chondroitin Sulfate, and the Two in Combination for Painful Knee Osteoarthritis."

Guo, et al, "Hawthorn Extract for Treating Chronic Heart Failure (Review)."

Moertl, et al, "Dose-Dependent Effects of Omega-3-Polyunsaturated Fatty Acids."

Mortenson, et al, "The Effect of Coenzyme Q10 on Morbidity and Mortality in Chronic Heart Failure."

Pavelká, et al, "Glucosamine Sulfate Use and Delay of Progression of Knee Osteoarthritis."

Reginster, et al, "Long-Term Effects of Glucosamine Sulphate on Osteoarthritis Progression."

Wahner-Roedler, et al, "Dietary Soy Supplement on Fibromyalgia Symptoms."

Wahner-Roedler, et al, "The Effect of Grape Seed Extract on Estrogen Levels of Postmenopausal Women."

Xin, et al, "Effects of Fish Oil Supplementation on Cardiac Function in Chronic Heart Failure."

Zick, et al, "Hawthorn Extract Randomized Blinded Chronic Heart Failure (HERB CHF) Trial."

Lecture 4 Transcript

Supplements in Practice

Now that we've talked a bit about the pros and cons of supplements, let's take a closer look at some of the supplements I use in my integrative medicine practice at Mayo. As with almost all of the therapies we'll discuss in this series, supplements are rarely a substitute for conventional medical treatment, and they're almost never a stand-alone solution. In other words, first build your N.E.S.S. foundation—nutrition, exercise, stress management, and social support. Then, and only then, if you still have a persisting symptom or a problem, talk to your health-care team if you're considering adding a supplement in a targeted and evidence-based fashion.

And remember what we mean by integrative: With integrative medicine, the idea is to integrate treatments that complement whatever conventional treatment your doctor may recommend—because conventional medicine is not standing still. The most effective use of supplements, or of any other complementary therapy, may change as advances are made on the more conventional side of medicine. That's why you and your doctor need to take an active role in evaluating and reevaluating your treatment, taking into account whatever new medications and treatments may become available, and how well they fit with elements of your existing treatment plan.

For example, I mentioned earlier that some patients are interested in trying glucosamine for arthritis pain. Many of us are troubled by knee pain, particularly the athletes among us. Because the cartilage inside our knees doesn't have a great blood supply, it often doesn't heal well after injury. That led several groups of researchers to explore the possibility of actually regrowing the cartilage. If they succeed, making it possible to treat the cause of pain directly with new cartilage, there won't be much need for a pain-easing supplement.

But in the meantime, glucosamine may provide some relief. Glucosamine is one the most widely used dietary supplements—you may have tried it yourself. Our bodies naturally make glucosamine, which is an amino sugar. Glucosamine supplements sold in stores are typically made from the skeletons of shellfish, and there are several forms. The form best suited for cartilage repair appears to be glucosamine sulfate.

Study results on glucosamine for cartilage repair have varied—partly because not all of the studies have used the same type of glucosamine, and because not all of the studies included a placebo comparison or ensured that neither the patient nor the researchers knew which pill was being administered. That said, several studies show that glucosamine sulfate is helpful in treating osteoarthritis. One study found that it improved symptoms of osteoarthritis, while another study showed that it improved symptoms of osteoarthritis-related pain, function, and stiffness by up to 25%. A more recent meta-analysis that looked at 17 published trials concluded that glucosamine sulfate might delay the progression and help symptoms of knee osteoarthritis.

People with osteoarthritis use supplements such as glucosamine in hopes that the supplement can improve their symptoms and reduce their need for pain-relieving medications—such as nonsteroidal anti-inflammatory drugs, or NSAIDs—which can be more expensive and may cause serious side effects. Glucosamine is often taken together with chondroitin, which also comes from cartilage—usually cow and shark cartilage. It's not clear if combining the two compounds is more effective than taking them alone. Studies looking at both glucosamine and chondroitin are mixed. The products appear to be safe and to produce fewer side effects than many other medications, but people who are allergic to shellfish should avoid them, however. Early studies of these supplements produced very promising results, but a few recent studies question whether these supplements can actually make a difference.

Here's an example: A study in the *New England Journal of Medicine* looked at about 1500 people with osteoarthritis of the knee. Over a period of 24 weeks, some individuals took glucosamine, some took chondroitin, and some took both supplements. Others in the study took a placebo or the medication celecoxib, sold as Celebrex, which is used to treat osteoarthritis.

The results showed that those who took glucosamine, chondroitin, or a combination of the two didn't notice any improvement in symptoms compared to those who only took the placebo. Only the participants who took the medication experienced a significant improvement, compared to placebo.

But this study was far from perfect. In fact, one of the key challenges critics have noted is that the participants taking the placebo itself actually had a 60% response rate. That's an extremely high placebo response, and it means that glucosamine and chondroitin would have had to had an even higher response rate to be rated as that effective. However, even given this limitation, when the researchers looked at the subset of participants who actually had really bad osteoarthritis, 79% of them who took the combined supplements actually did see improvement. It's unfortunate that a very expensive trial seems to have left us with as many questions as when we started.

So here's what I tell my patients: I don't have anything in my conventional pharmaceutical toolkit that might improve or repair cartilage. With that said, glucosamine and chondroitin are generally safe and may offer some relief to some people with osteoarthritis—at least some studies seem to suggest this. So along with N.E.S.S. as the foundation, I'll often have my patients try glucosamine and chondroitin, and I usually ask them to stay on it for 3–4 months before they decide if it's helpful or not. I'd estimate that a little more than half of my patients decide that they're getting some benefit from it and choose to stay on the combination indefinitely. For those who haven't seen any improvement after 4 months, we explore other options.

As with other types of supplements, a major issue is product quality. There's a lot of variability among glucosamine plus chondroitin supplements. In the past, some products contained no chondroitin despite label claims, while others contained more chondroitin than the label showed. And price isn't always a guarantee of quality. But again, with the current good manufacturing rules now in place, I think finding quality supplements is getting easier.

Another supplement that may be useful in treating arthritis is SAMe, which is short for S-adenosyl-L-methionine, a naturally occurring chemical in the human body that helps produce and regulate many hormones. A synthetic version of SAMe has become a popular dietary supplement in the United States, used for arthritis, depression, and liver disease. SAMe has been studied extensively in the treatment of osteoarthritis. Multiple trials indicate that it can relieve pain from arthritis as effectively as non-steroidal anti-inflammatory drugs, or NSAIDs, but with fewer side effects. However, it may take up to 30 days to get significant relief.

Clinical trials have suggested that SAMe can also improve symptoms of fibromyalgia, which can cause chronic pain as well as depressive symptoms. SAMe isn't approved by the FDA to treat depression in the United States, but it's used in Europe as a prescription drug to treat depression. SAMe may be helpful, but more research is needed. It isn't recommended for people with bipolar disorder because it may trigger mania. SAMe can enhance the action of the serotonin reuptake blockers that are commonly used to treat depression, so it's important not to combine the drugs, except under a doctor's supervision. SAMe can also interact with other drugs or supplements to affect blood pressure, blood glucose, or the risk of bleeding, so be sure your doctor is aware of everything you're taking. The bottom line is that you have to weigh the pros and cons. If the supplement you want to take is generally safe for your situation, you can try it for a month or two and see if you notice any improvement in symptoms. If you're not noticing a difference, stop taking it.

In our parents' generation, aches and pains may have been considered a normal part of aging. But these days, almost nothing about aging Is accepted without question. Most everyone would like to look or, at least, feel young. For many women, hormones became part of their medical vocabulary in the early '80s, when doctors routinely began using hormone therapy—the hormone estrogen taken alone or combined with hormone progesterone—to treat symptoms of menopause. The therapy was part of the Women's Health Initiative, which began in 1991 and involved more than

160,000 generally healthy, post-menopausal women. Clinical trials were designed to test the effects of postmenopausal hormone therapy, as well as changes in diet and calcium and vitamin D on heart disease, fractures, and breast and colorectal cancer.

At that time, doctors looked to hormones not only to treat hot flashes and night sweats but also to ease other symptoms that can come along with menopause. Hormones were used to help prevent bone loss, which happens when the body stops producing estrogen. Some studies also seemed to indicate that hormones might help protect the heart, and possibly prevent dementia. The use of hormone therapy changed abruptly when results released in 2002 from the Women's Health Initiative found that one type of hormone therapy actually increased more health risks than benefits, particularly when it was given to older, postmenopausal women. Trials found that combination estrogen-progestin pills increased the risks of heart disease, strokes, blood clots, and breast cancer.

As concerns about health hazards attributed to hormone therapy grew, doctors became less likely to prescribe it, and women were less inclined to take hormone therapy. The medical community backed away from hormone therapy use, and research kind of dropped off the radar. Today, hormone therapy is no longer recommended for disease prevention such as heart disease or memory loss. However, further review of clinical trials and new evidence shows that hormone therapy may be a good choice for certain women to treat hot flashes and sleep difficulties, depending on their risk factors. What all of this research shows is that use of hormone therapy to treat symptoms of menopause needs to be individualized. Hormones are not a one-size-fits-all treatment.

Many of my patients have asked about the safety of bioidentical hormones to treat symptoms of menopause. Bioidentical basically means that the hormones in the product are chemically the same as the ones in your body. But, in fact, the hormones in the bioidentical medications might not be any different than those in traditional hormone therapy. Because many bioidentical hormones are marketed as natural, people think they're safer, but they aren't. And there isn't any evidence that they're more effective. Natural only means the hormones come from plant or animal sources;

they're not synthesized in a lab. However, many of them still need to be commercially processed to become bioidentical.

Some people view bioidentical hormones as almost magical. But they carry the same risks as hormone therapy, and so you should definitely talk with your doctor before using them. For women with severe hot flashes that interfere with their quality of life, hormone therapy may be prescribed for a short period—maybe 3–5 years, and possibly longer if your doctor feels prolonged use would be safe. So are there any supplements we can offer our patients as they move through this phase of their lives?

Black cohosh, a member of the buttercup family, is a plant that was used in Native American medicine and was a home remedy for rheumatism and arthritis in 19th-century America. The underground stems and roots of black cohosh are commonly used fresh or dried to make strong teas known as infusions, capsules, extracts used in pills, or liquid extracts—also called tinctures. In recent years, black cohosh has become popular for treating hot flashes, night sweats, vaginal dryness, and other symptoms of menopause. Black cohosh also has been used for menstrual irregularities, and premenstrual syndrome, and to induce labor.

Black cohosh drew attention as an herbal remedy for hot flashes and other menopausal symptoms after hormone replacement therapy fell out of favor, and anecdotal reports and small trials of black cohosh seemed promising. But a meta-analysis of six double-blind, randomized, clinical trials for relief of menopausal symptoms found that black cohosh—whether used alone or with other botanicals—failed to relieve hot flashes and night sweats in postmenopausal women or those approaching menopause.

For the most part, clinical trials of black cohosh to treat menopausal symptoms haven't found that the herb causes serious side effects, but some people taking black cohosh have experienced stomach discomfort, headache, or rash. There's also been case reports of the liver disease—such as hepatitis—as well as liver failure, in some women who took black cohosh. Although these cases are rare, and the evidence isn't definitive, scientists are still concerned about how the herb may affect the liver. If you take birth control pills, hormone replacement therapy, sedatives, or blood pressure medication, don't take black cohosh without your doctor's approval. My take: Since hot flashes can be a difficult symptom to treat, I'm open to having my patients do a trial of black cohosh, especially if they haven't had success with conventional approaches.

Soy is another plant that has been traditionally used to treat menopausal symptoms—as well as osteoporosis, memory problems, high blood pressure, high cholesterol levels, breast cancer and prostate cancer. Soy has been common in Asian diets for thousands of years and is found in modern American diets as a food or food additive. As a dietary supplement, soy is available in tablets and in capsules that may contain isoflavones or phytoestrogens, soy protein, or both.

Some studies suggest that soy isoflavone supplements may reduce hot flashes in women after menopause, but the results have been inconsistent. There's not enough scientific evidence to know if soy supplements are effective for any other health uses. Although the American Heart Association says that eating soy-based food doesn't significantly lower cholesterol, some research suggests that daily intake of soy protein may slightly lower levels of low-density lipoprotein—also known as LDL or bad cholesterol.

Most people can consume soy safely as a food or for short periods as a dietary supplement. You may experience minor nausea, bloating, and constipation with soy. In rare cases, allergic reactions such as breathing problems and a rash could occur. We don't know yet how safe soy isoflavones are when they're taken long term. Evidence is mixed on whether using isoflavone supplements over time can increase the risk of endometrial hyperplasia, a thickening of the lining of the uterus that could lead to cancer. Dietary soy, on the other hand, doesn't seem to affect the risk of this condition.

Soy's possible role in breast cancer risk is uncertain. Until we know more about soy's effect on estrogen levels, women with breast cancer or who have a higher risk of developing breast cancer should be careful about using soy and should discuss its use with their health care providers. My take: In general, eating soy foods seems safe and may be beneficial.

Taking high doses of soy supplements, on the other hand, doesn't seem to have a lot of proven benefits and may lead to some risks.

Men have their own difficulties at this time of life, and many of you likely know someone who struggles with an enlarged prostate gland. Saw palmetto has been used as an alternative treatment for the urinary symptoms associated with an enlarged prostate—also called benign prostatic hyperplasia, or BPH. It's also taken for chronic pelvic pain, bladder disorders, decreased sex drive, hair loss, hormone imbalances, and prostate cancer. Saw palmetto is a small palm tree native to the eastern United States. Supplements made from saw palmetto are available as liquid extracts, tablets, capsules, and as an infusion or a tea.

Several small studies suggest that saw palmetto may be effective for treating BPH symptoms, but a 2011 study of 369 older men showed that saw palmetto didn't reduce BPH-related urinary symptoms more than placebo—an inactive substance. Earlier studies produced similar results. Again, my take: BPH is such a vexing problem for so many men as they age. Many conventional medicines to treat it are expensive or can have side effects, so I often have my patients try saw palmetto to see if they get any positive results. I usually recommend it in a combination product that contains other herbs like stinging nettle, beta-sitosterol and pumpkin seed. Since different herbs may be working via different mechanisms, this is one instance in which a combination product may have some advantages. At the same time, many of my patients use saw palmetto and get good results. This is one of those times in which keeping a good record of your response to a supplement can really help you determine which one may be right for you.

So far we've talked about common complaints of aging, but it may surprise you to know that supplements may also play a role in treatment of more complicated, life-threatening conditions like heart disease. When we think of heart disease, most of us naturally first think about the dramatic events surrounding a heart attack. There's no question; if you're experiencing a heart attack, the best thing you can do is take advantage of the modern technology that conventional medicine has to offer. This means getting to the hospital as quickly as possible, probably having an angiogram, and maybe getting a stent placed, or even undergoing open-heart surgery. To be honest, integrative medicine has very little to offer in the midst of that dramatic and time-critical series of events. Where integrative medicine may have some impact is on the prevention of that catastrophic event in the first place, and perhaps in dealing with the sequelae.

When it comes to preventing heart disease, it's not possible to overstate the importance of the four principles of N.E.S.S.—nutrition, exercise, stress management, and social support—that we've been discussing throughout this course as an overall strategy for optimizing health and wellness.

When we think about the sequelae of heart disease—the negative aftereffects—one of the more challenging for many patients is something called congestive heart failure, or CHF. The terminology is a bit confusing. In my mind, when I hear the word failure, it makes me think of something that's not working at all. But in reality, congestive heart failure simply means that the heart muscle is no longer pumping as effectively as it once did. So even though it has significant risks and can lead to death, heart failure is perhaps a bit of an ominous name for something that many patients face after having heart damage from a heart attack.

Again, the good news is that conventional medicine has a number of treatments—such as beta blockers and ACE inhibitors—that have been shown to reduce the risk of further heart disease and help alleviate the symptoms of heart failure. In some cases, they may even help to remodel the heart muscle back into a nearly normal function. So, as with everything else in this course, you'll want to make sure that you're not neglecting or overlooking the importance of following the best conventional medical practices your care team can provide.

Once you've done that, is there anything in the integrative medicine room that might be helpful? When you look at Natural Medicines Comprehensive Database, which is compiled by a team of pharmacists and medical doctors, two supplements stand out: Coenzyme Q10 and fish oil. Let's take a look at coenzyme Q10 first.

Coenzyme Q10 is an antioxidant made by your body and used by cells throughout your body for their basic functions, with chemical structure 2,3-dimethoxy-5-methyl-6-decaprenyl-1,4-benzoquinone; it is sometimes even called ubiquinone because of its ubiquitous distribution throughout the human body. The coenzyme is concentrated in the mitochondria, the power plants of the cell, and plays a vital role in the production of chemical energy by participating in the production of adenosine triphosphate—or ATP—the body's so-called energy currency. Essentially, it helps your body convert food into energy. There have been a number of trials looking at the effects of coenzyme Q10 and congestive heart failure. Coenzyme Q10 has been shown to reduce mortality by nearly half in certain patients with moderate to severe heart failure.

Svend Mortensen, from the Heart Centre at Copenhagen University Hospital in Denmark, and his colleagues reported on a study in 2012 involving more than 400 patients in a long-term, double-blind, randomized placebo-controlled trial. With interventions of 100 milligrams of coenzyme Q10, 3 times a day, measured against the placebo, coenzyme Q10 significantly reduced the risk of major adverse cardiac events and mortality.

After 2 years, 25% of patients in the placebo group had a major adverse cardiovascular event compared to 14% in the study group. Mortality and hospitalizations were also lower in the study group. Over the 2-year period, 18 patients died in the coenzyme Q10 group—9%—compared to 36 patients, or 17%, in the placebo group.

The authors also look at potential mechanisms of action and found that the coenzyme Q10 decreased NT-proBNP—that's a laboratory finding that's associated with heart failure. BNP, or brain natriuretic peptide, is a small, ringed peptide secreted by the heart to regulate blood pressure and fluid balance. When it's stretched and working hard to pump blood, your heart produces and releases BNP and NT-proBNP. Dr. Mortensen concluded that these results made, in his words "a strong case for coenzyme Q10, a natural substance that's virtually without side effects, to be considered as part of the maintenance therapy for all patients with chronic heart failure."

At Tulane University, Dr. A. Domnica Fotino and her colleagues performed a meta-analysis in 2012 on the effect of coenzyme Q10 supplementation on chronic heart failure. They pooled studies going back to the early '80s, and then looked at all the data from each of them in aggregate. The analysis showed that coenzyme Q10 supplementation may be of benefit to patients with chronic heart failure, particularly those with less-severe cases. They found significant improvement in something called the ejection fraction—that's a measure of how well your heart is pumping, the percentage of blood leaving your heart each time it contracts.

These are just two of many trials out there, but I think you can see that coenzyme Q10 is something to talk about with your health-care team if you're dealing with congestive heart failure. It's important to note that in most of the studies on coenzyme Q10, it was used as an adjunct—that means it was used after the conventional therapy had already been in place. So, we should consider coenzyme Q10 as part of an overall strategy, not as a substitute for conventional therapy.

Another supplement that has shown effectiveness in treating congestive heart failure is fish oil, which is one of the most widely used dietary supplements in the United States. Using fish oil to promote good health isn't a new concept. Taking cod liver oil as a source of vitamin D first became popular in 19th-century England, and fish oil has been studied for heart health since it was found that the Inuit people of Greenland have a lower risk of heart disease even though they eat a high-fat diet. Fish oil contains two omega-3 fatty acids called docosahexaenoic acid, or DHA; and eicosapentaenoic acid, or EPA. Some nuts, seeds, and vegetable oils contain alpha-linolenic acid or ALA. When consumed, the ALA is converted to DHA or EPA. Compared to people in other nations with lower rates of heart disease, such as Japan, people in the United States tend to have less DHA and EPA in their bodies. Here's why this difference is important:

Studies have shown that the risk of congestive heart failure is lower in older adults who have higher levels of EPA. In one study of patients with congestive heart failure, those taking fish oil had better vasodilation and better peak oxygen consumption, as well as decreases in interleukin 6 and tumor necrosis factor—two common inflammatory agents. In a meta-analysis by Dr. Xin and colleagues in Beijing, the data from more than 800 patients, from 7 different trials, was analyzed. They concluded that using fish oil in supplements in patients with congestive heart failure resulted in a number of improvements in the overall function of the heart. Dr. Xin concluded that "Improvement in cardiac functioning, remodeling, and functional capacity may be important mechanisms underlying the therapeutic role of fish oil."

Keep in mind that high doses of fish oil can be harmful. Too much fish oil can increase your risk of bleeding, cause higher levels of low-density lipoprotein—LDL, or bad cholesterol—and also cause problems controlling your blood sugar. Many people ask me why we simply can't eat more fish, and I think that's part of an overall healthy nutrition strategy. However, there are ongoing concerns about fish and especially the accumulation of toxic chemicals, such as mercury, that make eating fish every day at least somewhat problematic.

One final supplement we should consider is hawthorn berries, which have been around for a long time, with a rather long history of efficacy for treating congestive heart failure. A specialized systematic review conducted by the Cochrane group looked at more than 850 patients from 10 different trials and concluded in 2008 that the use of hawthorn among patients with chronic heart failure resulted in improvement in maximum workload and exercise tolerance, and reduced symptoms with very few adverse effects. To sum up their findings, the researchers said—and I'll quote them here: "These results suggest a significant benefit in symptom control and physiologic outcomes from hawthorn extract as an adjunct of treatment for congestive heart failure."

So, at this point, things looked promising for hawthorn. But then Dr. Suzanna Zick and some of her colleagues at the University of Michigan published the results of a trial in 2009 that seemed to rebuke all of these positive encouraging trials. Dr. Zick's group monitored patients taking 450 milligrams of hawthorn, twice a day, for 6 months. Unlike previous studies, these researchers saw no improvement in exercise tolerance or peak oxygen consumption. That led them to conclude that hawthorn isn't helpful from a symptomatic or a functional standpoint when it's given with standard medical therapy for heart failure.

I've known Dr. Zick for many years, and know that she has a particular interest in herbal therapy and herbal research, so I was intrigued by the fact that she seemed to have obtained such contrary findings. I called her and asked why she thought her trial was so different from some of the older hawthorn trials that seemed to do so well. She noted that in many of the older trials, many of the patients were not on optimal conventional therapy. Some of the trials were also old enough that the optimal treatment of congestive heart failure had not yet been discovered. Thus, in patients who don't have access to the best of conventional medical management of congestive heart failure, hawthorn probably does have something to offer. But for most of us, if we're receiving the best conventional treatments available, it seems like hawthorn probably falls by the wayside. This brings us back to the point I raised at the beginning of this lecture: We need to continually re-evaluate complementary therapies in relation to changes in what conventional medicine has to offer.

So my approach when working with patients who have congestive heart failure, and who are interested in dietary supplements, is to tell them that it's reasonable to explore possibly using coenzyme Q10 and fish oil. I think the evidence on hawthorn is somewhat conflicting. Though it's likely safe, I don't think it offers much in the way of benefit; and I really don't want my patients taking more medications than they have to, whether they're natural or otherwise.

This brings me to one last principle: repletion. Whenever I see a patient with congestive heart failure, I always check the patient's vitamin D level as part of my workup. And if they're low on vitamin D, I put them on a vitamin D3 supplement. For individuals low in certain nutrients, supplements make sense. That doesn't mean that people whose vitamin D levels are already in the normal range would benefit from the same treatment.

We've looked at just a few conditions in this lecture, but I hope you get the idea: To be an educated consumer, you have to keep asking, "What makes sense for me today?" What worked for you at age 30 may not make sense for you at age 50, and conventional treatments may change as well. We need to view all medications—complementary and prescription—in the same light and see how well they work. It takes time and a thoughtful approach. In the next lecture, we'll take a look at a type of complementary therapy that doesn't involve minerals, vitamins, hormones, or any type of pill. All you need is an open mind.

Lecture 5

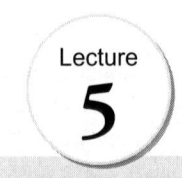

Mind-Body Medicine

Mind-body medicine focuses on how the power of your thought process can change what's happening in your body. You can't wish cancer away, but you can help train your attention. And by training your attention, you can address anxiety and even work to create new pathways that help you experience less stress and anger. In this lecture, you will learn about some of the great ways that mind-body practices can be used as part of your overall health and wellness plan.

The Power of the Mind

- The power and speed of the mind is phenomenal. Let's take the stress response and the relaxation response as an example. The stress response is the fight-or-flight response; it automatically kicks in when you're faced with danger. Your body pumps up your heart rate, increases blood flow to your muscles, and decreases blood flow to the parts of your body that aren't needed to face the threat.

- The opposite of the stress response is the relaxation response. It's something that takes practice, but through approaches such as practicing meditation or deep breathing, you can train your body in a way that slows down your heart rate and breathing and increases your focus on the present moment. The way your mind can work in these two instances tells us a lot about the power of the mind-body connection—and makes mind-body medicine a fascinating area of medical study.

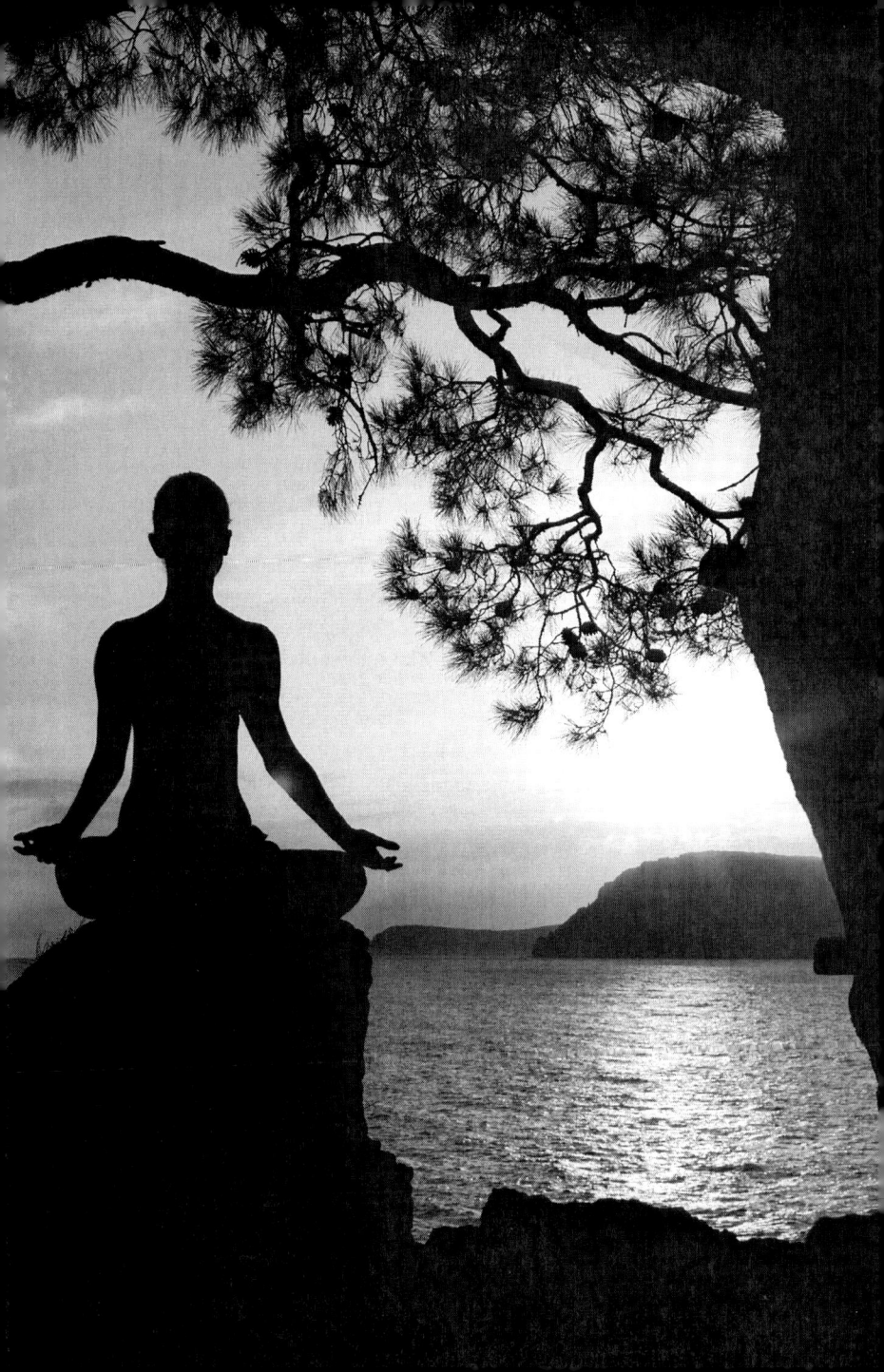

- Mind-body practices have two core components.

    1. Restore the mind to a state of peaceful neutrality. In this state, your mind achieves a state that's nonjudgmental, efficient, and adaptive to your needs. To reach this state, the mind has to shed negative experiences acquired over the years.

    2. Once your mind is "ready," use it in ways that help you achieve good health. This might be through spiritual intervention or prayer, a spoken intervention such as transcendental meditation, or through practices that involve breathing and posture or soothing imagery.

- As we learn newer and more refined mind-body techniques, it's important to recognize the simplicity of their underlying concepts. At their core, mind-body interventions are based on the values of peace, forgiveness, sharing, selflessness, integrity, and love—values that can help you achieve the outcomes you seek.

- Chronic stress may lead to genetic changes that increase the amount of inflammation in our body. Chronic stress can do all kinds of terrible things to our cardiovascular systems, from raising the risk of hypertension, to increasing the risk of heart attacks, to making blood vessels less pliable.

- It's time for us to recognize that what happens to us mentally or emotionally can have a profound impact on our health. And it's worth noting that if you even simply *think* about something bad, your body will start to prepare just like it's actually happening.

- Fortunately, we can harness that same imaginative power for our good. Just like thinking about something stressful may have negative physiologic effects, the reverse of that—the relaxation response—can induce positive effects in our body.

- This is where practices such as meditation, guided imagery, or even yoga or tai chi—things that can help calm the brain—become a great tool in our approach to optimize our health and wellness.

- A simple approach is to think about a quiet space or place. You could imagine, for example, the last time you were at a beach—and by slowing your breathing and focusing on that pleasant memory, you can start to raise your heart rate variability (which has been shown to improve health overall) and lower your stress response.

Neuroplasticity and Mind-Body Practices

- While the stress response is good for life-threatening situations, most of us face few truly life-threatening situations each day. That means that we're overreacting to the various small stressors we face each day.

- Our brains are hardwired to keep reusing the responses we have in place. So, if you respond in a fight-or-flight way to a small stressor, that's how your brain will automatically respond to a small stressor the next time you experience one. The good news is that you can train your brain to take a different path.

- That's where neuroplasticity comes in. Neuroplasticity means that the brain is "plastic," or changeable, and that we can retrain it to react in more skillful ways. Mind-body practitioners focus on two processes within the mind that together help craft your everyday experiences: attention and interpretation.

- The process of attention helps you screen, select, and absorb sensory information from the world. This information is then subject to interpretation, a process that relies on previous experience, preferences, and how you planned for things to go.

- The way you attend to the world around you can predispose you to stress, which can lead to illness. If you are constantly attending to what's wrong in the world, or in yourself, or in other people, you're interpreting your world in a mostly negative way.

- You're also likely to exaggerate those negative thoughts, so small irritations become large threats, and you feel chronically anxious and stressed. You may develop a rigid outlook that can get in the way of your ability to see things from a more mature perspective, which takes other viewpoints and outcomes into consideration.

- Mind-body therapists call this situation "mindlessness," and it's not good for your brain. In a state of mindlessness, you become disengaged from the real world and focused mainly on your anxiety-provoking thoughts. A mindless state not only invites stress, sleeplessness, and decreased quality of life, but also may predispose you to multiple medical conditions, some of them potentially life-threatening.

- The purpose of mind-body medicine is to help free you from excessive negative thoughts and the related state of mindlessness. The hope is to bring your attention to the present moment in a state of acceptance that empowers you to engage in meaningful action.

- In place of those negative thoughts, mind-body medicine is intended to help you cultivate transformative principles, such as forgiveness, acceptance, compassion, gratitude, interconnectedness, and a higher meaning to life. These principles can provide you with balanced optimism and openness to experience. They can help you see the reality—or lack thereof—in your thoughts.

- Amit Sood, M.D., who chairs the Mind-Body Medicine Initiative in Mayo Clinic's Complementary and Integrative Medicine Program, has found that small meditative practices—done three or four times a day for a few minutes each time—significantly reduces stress and slows breathing. For example, when you get out of bed and put your feet on the floor first thing in the morning, think of five things or people that you're grateful for and think kind thoughts or put forward good intentions. This doesn't rise to the level of deep meditation, but it can set the tone for your day.

- Dr. Sood also introduced the SMART (Stress Management and Resiliency Training) program, which is scientifically proven to decrease symptoms of stress and anxiety and increase well-being, resilience, self-regulation, mindfulness, happiness, and positive health behavior.

- Participants in the SMART program learn how to train their attention so that it is stronger and more focused in the present moment. They learn to guide their thoughts based on higher principles rather than by prejudices. The program has been tested in 10 completed research studies in and outside of Mayo Clinic, with the results showing a decrease in stress and anxiety and an improvement in positive health behaviors.

Biofeedback

- One way to start the rerouting process is through biofeedback, which is a technique you can use to learn to control your body's functions, such as your heart rate. With biofeedback, you're connected to electrical sensors that help you receive information about your body. This feedback helps you focus on making subtle changes in your body, such as relaxing certain muscles, to achieve the results you want, such as reducing pain.

- In essence, biofeedback gives you the power to use your thoughts to control your body, often to improve a health condition or your physical performance. Biofeedback is often used as a relaxation technique.

- Biofeedback, sometimes called biofeedback training, is used to help manage many physical and mental health issues, including the following.

o Anxiety or stress	o Constipation
o Asthma	o High blood pressure
o Chemotherapy side effects	o Incontinence
o Chronic pain	o Irritable bowel syndrome

- Although you can receive biofeedback training in physical therapy clinics, medical centers, and hospitals, more and more biofeedback devices and programs are being marketed for use at home. Some of these are handheld portable devices, while others connect to your computer. You can try different devices until you find one that works for you, or ask your doctor for advice. You might also check with your health insurance company to see what costs, if any, associated with biofeedback devices are covered.

- Two of the main types of equipment used in biofeedback are as follows.

  1. A breathing sensor monitors your breathing, helping you learn to breathe more slowly and deeply. It has also been shown to reduce blood pressure.

  2. A heart rate variability monitor shows the increases and decreases in your heart's natural cycle or rhythm. These devices measure the pulse in your fingertip or earlobe and display the time between your heartbeats. By controlling your breathing—more deeply and slowly—you can change your heart rate.

- For some people, biofeedback devices like these help produce a deep state of relaxation. Other people rely on practices such as meditation but use biofeedback devices to assess their progress.

And then other people find the devices distracting. You have to find what works for you.

- The following are four main types of biofeedback techniques for stress management and how they work.

    1. Electromyography biofeedback (EMG) gives you information about the tension of your muscles to help you practice relaxation.

    2. With temperature, or thermal, biofeedback, sensors attached to your fingers or feet measure your skin temperature and the blood flow to your skin. Because your temperature often drops when you're under stress, a low reading may prompt you to begin relaxation techniques.

    3. In galvanic skin response training, sensors measure the activity of your sweat glands and the amount of sweat on your skin, alerting you to anxiety.

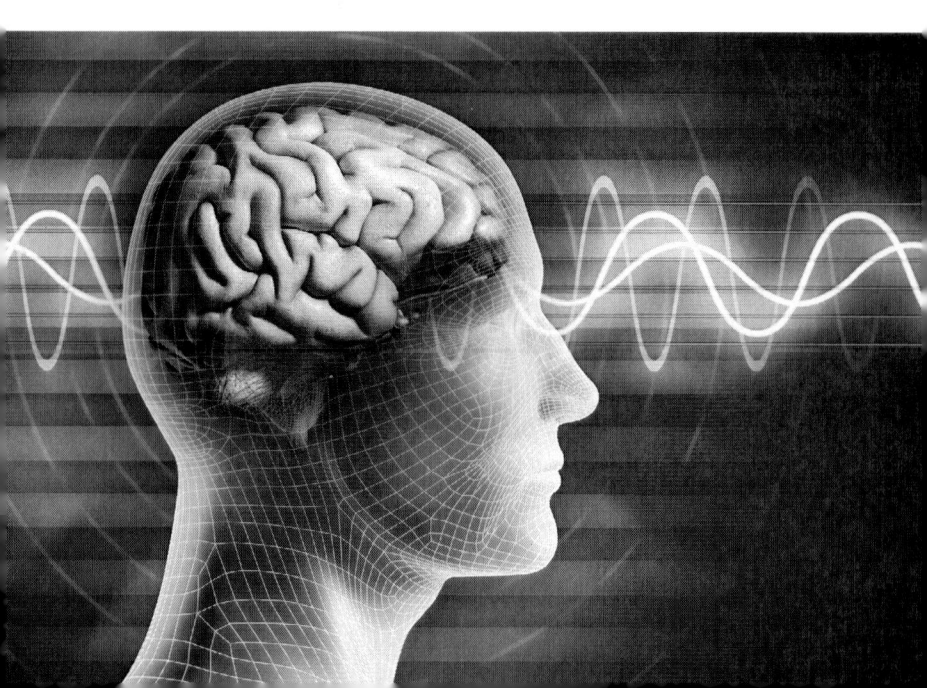

4. Heart rate variability biofeedback helps you control your heart rate in an effort to improve blood pressure, lung function, and stress and anxiety.

- If you're interested in trying biofeedback, the first step is to find a registered therapist. Start by asking your doctor or another health-care professional who's knowledgeable about biofeedback therapy to recommend someone who has experience in treating your condition.

- State laws regulating biofeedback practitioners vary. Many biofeedback therapists are licensed in another area of health care, such as nursing or physical therapy, and might work under the guidance of a doctor. Some biofeedback therapists choose to become certified to show that they have extra training and experience in the practice.

- When you find a potential biofeedback therapist, the following are some questions to ask before starting treatment.

    o Are you licensed, certified, or registered?

    o If you aren't licensed, are you working under the supervision of a licensed health-care professional?

    o What is your training and experience?

    o Do you have experience providing feedback for my condition?

    o How many biofeedback sessions do you think I'll need?

    o What is the cost, and is it covered by health insurance?

    o Can you provide a list of references?

Suggested Reading

Bays, *How to Train a Wild Elephant*.

Chesak, et al, "Enhancing Resilience among New Nurses."

Cutshall, et al, "Evaluation of a Biofeedback-Assisted Meditation Program as a Stress Management Tool."

Flugel Colle, et al, "Measurement of Quality of Life and Participant Experience."

Sharma, et al, "Bibliotherapy to Decrease Stress and Anxiety."

Sood, *The Mayo Clinic Guide to Stress-Free Living*.

———, *The Mayo Clinic Handbook for Happiness*.

Sood, et al, "Stress Management and Resiliency Training (SMART) Program."

U.S. Department of Health and Human Services, "Neuroplasticity."

Waller, et al, "Unresolved Trauma in Fibromyalgia."

Lecture 5 Transcript

Mind-Body Medicine

In the next few lectures, I'll address the mind-body connection and different mind-body practices you can try. When we say mind-body medicine, we're talking about how the power of your thought process can change what's happening in your body. You can't wish cancer away or think hard enough so that your diabetes disappears, but you can help train your attention. And by training your attention, you can address anxiety, and even work to create new pathways that help you experience less stress and anger.

These approaches aren't magic, and they aren't a miracle cure; but with practice and patience, they do help. My colleague Dr. Amit Sood, who oversees the mind-body initiative at Mayo Clinic, has a great way of summing up mind-body medicine: He says that mind-body medicine comes down to positively influencing the mind to improve the health of the individual. Let's talk about how mind-body medicine came to be.

The belief that mind and body are intricately connected goes back centuries. For most of our history, both scientists and laypeople never doubted that the mind and body were intertwined. But with the development of Western medicine during the 17th century, this basic connected approach to health and wellness sort of fell by the wayside. As scientists explored the inner workings of the human body with increasing fascination, they discovered and introduced such fundamental concepts as germs as a source of disease; and medications, like antibiotics, and surgical techniques as a way to treat disease—practices that remain central components of modern medicine.

However, treating disease strictly on a biological level has its limitations, as reflected by the growing number of individuals turning to treatments outside of modern medicine. Today, we're faced with several diseases, such as fibromyalgia and irritable bowel syndrome, that aren't curable with potent drugs or surgical procedures. This recognition—along with mounting scientific evidence pointing to the mind as one of several factors in the development of disease—has led to a resurgence of mind-body medicine. It has also increased interest in holistic health and healing, a practice that addresses the whole person—mind, body, and spirit—and brings together both conventional and alternative therapies in an effort to prevent disease, treat disease, and promote optimal health.

So now, in the last 20 or 30 years, we've seen a growing body of research that reaffirms the importance of the mind-body connection. Practitioners are using research findings to help people be healthier by recognizing how the mind affects the body and vice versa, how the body affects the mind. The power and speed of the mind is phenomenal. Let's take the stress response and relaxation response—which we talked about earlier in this course—as an example. The stress response is the fight or flight response; it automatically kicks in when you're faced with danger. Your body pumps up your heart rate, increases blood flow to your muscles, and decreases blood flow to the parts of your body that aren't needed to face the threat.

The opposite of the stress response is the relaxation response. It's something that takes practice, but through approaches such as practicing meditation or deep breathing, you can train your body in a way that slows down your heart rate and your breathing, and increases your focus on the present moment. The way your mind can work in these two instances tells us a lot about the power of the mind-body connection and makes mind-body medicine a fascinating area of medical study. An intriguing part of mind-body medicine, which is undergoing increasing study, is how mind and body respond to the healing effect of other minds. The positive benefits of interventions, such as a support group, may relate in part to the comfort and sense of security that comes with being part of a tribe. We'll talk about that more; later, when we address spirituality.

Mind-body practices have two core components: One, restore the mind to a state of peaceful neutrality. In this state, your mind achieves a state that's nonjudgmental, efficient, and adaptive to your needs. To reach this state, the mind has to shed negative experiences acquired over the years.

Two, once your mind is ready, use it in ways that help you achieve good health. This might be through spiritual intervention or prayer, a spoken intervention such as transcendental meditation, or through practices that involve breathing and posture, or soothing imagery.

As we learn newer and more refined mind-body techniques, it's important to recognize the simplicity of their underlying concepts. At their core, mind-body interventions are based on the values of peace, forgiveness, sharing, selflessness, integrity, and love—values that can help you achieve the outcomes you seek.

A powerful testament to the power of the mind-body connection is in the study of trauma. Studies show that many people who experience fibromyalgia may have had a traumatic event somewhere in their past. And more generally, for many people, a history of abuse is often a factor in how the brain develops. How could something that happened 10 or 15 years ago now manifest as widespread body pain, chronic fatigue, brain fog, and so on? We are just beginning to understand how trauma can lead to rewiring of the brain and have an ongoing impact on our health.

As we think about the effects of stress, it becomes a bit easier to see the connection. For example, we know that wounds tend to heal more slowly in people who are under chronic stress. In other people, stress may cause the immune system to not work as well. And we know that people under chronic stress have a less robust response to the flu vaccine. Chronic stress may also lead to genetic changes that actually increase the amount of inflammation in our body. Of course, I think it's pretty widely recognized that chronic stress can do all sorts of terrible things to our cardiovascular systems, from raising the risk of high blood pressure, to increasing the risk of heart attacks, to making blood vessels less pliable.

The point is, it's high time for us to recognize that what happens to us mentally or emotionally can have a profound impact on our health. And it's worth noting that if you even simply think about something bad, your body will start to prepare just like it's actually happening. So just thinking about the IRS audit that may or may not happen could cause your adrenal glands to release adrenaline and start a cascade of effects from the simple thought of a stressful event. Fortunately, we can harness that same imaginative power for our good. Just like thinking about something stressful may have negative physiologic effects, the reverse of that—the relaxation response that I mentioned earlier—can actually induce positive effects in our body.

This is where practices such as meditation, guided imagery, or even yoga or tai chi—things that can help calm the brain—become a great tool in our approach to optimize our health and wellness. For me, a simple approach is to think about a quiet space or place. You could imagine, for example, the last time you were at a beach. And by slowing your breathing and focusing on that pleasant memory, you can actually start to raise your heart rate variability and lower your stress response.

Heart rate variability—slight variations in the timing of each heartbeat—reflects an ongoing balancing act between the sympathetic and parasympathetic parts of our autonomic nervous system. When your sympathetic nervous system is predominant, it tends to make the heart rate variability go down, and your heart rate becomes like a metronome. When you have a good balance with your parasympathetic system, there's more variability because one system is urging the heart beat to go faster, while the other's working to slow it down. Higher variability means there's a more active balance between the two systems, and this has been shown to improve health overall.

So, if you take time regularly for a relaxation exercise like the one I just described, you can begin to quiet down your sympathetic response, the part of your nervous system that triggers an all-hands-on-deck, crisis response to a stressor; and raise your parasympathetic response, that part of your nervous system that causes relaxation.

How do I approach mind-body medicine with my patients? If they're seeing me for a check-up or to talk about how to improve their health and wellness, I start by talking about the Dean Ornish study we addressed in the very first lecture—how working on nutrition, exercise, stress management, and support all affect your very chromosomes, the telomeres.

If they have a chronic condition, we talk about an overall health plan and why they should be engaged in mind-body approaches. People are very responsive because we're not couching it in a woo-woo kind of Eastern mysticism. We talk about what the research has found, and on a scientific level, what chronic stress can do in terms of brain volume and neurologic responsiveness. We talk about the prefrontal cortex, which is critical for executive functioning like setting goals, monitoring progress toward those goals, and focusing attention. The prefrontal cortex tends to shrink with age and under stress, and those abilities correspondingly decline, so training the brain is an important part of the health process.

When I talk to patients about stress, most of them simply don't realize its impact. Most patients are pretty quick to know their cholesterol numbers or blood pressure, but they don't recognize the degree to which high levels of stress have become part of their daily lives. Most are over-scheduled and multitasking right up to when they go to bed. Many of them don't have extended families nearby or a close connection to a church or synagogue.

So they're experiencing unprecedented levels of daily, chronic stress. And all the while, at the same time, society as a whole has largely minimized the role of family and religious connections in our lives. With nowhere to unload, many of my patients turn to overeating, drinking, or taking up casual relationships as ways of dealing with the stress—the very same stress that most of them don't even recognize they have. They often don't see how their own maladaptive behaviors can be causing health problems, too. With this in mind, I start the conversation with the idea that it's important to address stress responses—whether it's flipping someone off in traffic or shouting at your spouse.

While the stress response is good for life-threatening situations, most of us face few truly life-threatening situations each day. That means that we're overreacting to the 101 little stressors we face each day. It's also important to recognize that our brains are hardwired to keep reusing the responses we have in place. So if you respond in a fight or flight kind of way to a small stressor, that's how your brain will automatically respond to a small stressor the next time you experience one. The good news is that you can train your brain to take a different path.

That's where neuroplasticity comes in. Neuroplasticity means that the brain is plastic or changeable, and that we can retrain it to react in more skillful ways. Mind-body practitioners focus on two processes within the mind that together help craft your everyday experiences: attention and interpretation.

The process of attention helps you screen, select, and absorb sensory information from the world. This information is then subject to interpretation, a process that relies on previous experience, preferences, and how you planned for things to go. The way you attend to the world around you can predispose you to stress, which can lead to illness. If you are constantly attending to what's wrong in the world, or in yourself, or other people, you're interpreting your world in a mostly negative way.

You're also likely to exaggerate those negative thoughts so that small irritations become large threats, and you feel chronically anxious and stressed. You may develop a rigid outlook—that won't work, or that never happens. This can get in the way of your ability to see things from a more mature perspective, which takes other viewpoints and outcomes into consideration. Mind-body therapists call this situation mindlessness, and we already know it's not good for your brain.

In a state of mindlessness, you become disengaged from the real world and what it's really like, and focus mainly on your anxiety-provoking thoughts. A mindless state not only invites stress, sleeplessness, and decreased quality of life; but also may predispose you to multiple medical conditions, some of them potentially life-threatening. This is where the concept of mind-body medicine comes in. The purpose of mind-body medicine is to help free you from excessive negative thoughts and the related state of mindlessness. The hope is to bring your attention to the present moment in a state of acceptance that empowers you to engage in meaningful action.

In place of those negative thoughts, mind-body medicine is intended to help you cultivate transformative principles, like forgiveness, acceptance, compassion, gratitude, interconnectedness, and a higher meaning to life. These principles can provide you with balanced optimism and openness to experience. They can help you see the reality, or lack thereof, in your thoughts.

Let's talk a little bit more about neuroplasticity—the ability of the brain to grow and change throughout the lifespan. As we just learned, when we're retraining the brain, we're addressing attention and interpretation. We're creating new ways of paying attention, and opening ourselves up to different ways of thinking—maybe that person who cut you off in traffic is on the way to the hospital to get to a loved one who's been in a tragic accident. With compassion in mind, how does your body react? Do you feel and react differently knowing that information? Or do you still react with that same anger?

By creating these new routes in your brain and driving along them again and again, you can lower your stress level and work on principles that will help give your life deeper meaning. The concept of neuroplasticity is fairly new. It wasn't that long ago, or perhaps it was, when I was a medical student. At that time, the general thinking was that we had a set number of neurons in our brains. With age, we thought, not much good could happen to the neurons in our brains, but a lot of bad things were likely—such as shrinkage of the brain, or loss of those neural connections, and, of course, conditions like Alzheimer's.

However, a lot of research in the last 10 or 15 years has helped us understand that the brain is not static; it has a great deal of neuroplasticity. Really, up to any age, we can actually create new connections in our brains. This seems to happen best when we do a lot of positive things for overall health, such as optimizing nutrition—perhaps emphasizing more berries in our diet—maintaining good aerobic exercise or activity, connecting socially with others, and creating novelty for our brain on a regular basis.

Even in older individuals, such an approach has been shown to slow the loss of neurons and brain connections, and in some cases enhance or even restore much of that function. For a long time, we heard that doing crosswords or putting puzzles together would help keep your brain active. But the trick is to keep mixing it up, like you do for your exercise routine. Once you start doing crosswords, your brain gets used to it; so every three months, try something new—learn a new language, try a new hobby. In essence, do something different to engage and interest your brain.

Let me give you an example of how we practice this at Mayo Clinic: Dr. Sood, whom I mentioned earlier in this lecture, came here from India. He realized that most Americans have lost the ability to focus their attention, and asking someone to sit and be still and quiet for 20, 40, or 60 minutes was almost impossible.

Another issue he found was that people tended to connect meditation to religion. Meditation is a part of most major religions, and this caused some problems for some people who saw meditation as something you did with a guru in India. For example, they thought that meditation was Eastern and had to be embedded in a religion like Hinduism. They didn't understand that meditation has been transformed into a practice featuring universal elements—focused attention and slowed breathing, for example—but without a religious connection. We know that the benefits of meditation are universal, so making it a secular practice, while honoring its main components, has been a key strategy in making meditation available to anyone who wants to explore it.

With all of this in mind, Dr. Sood thought, "How can we strip away the religious component and focus on the essential parts of meditation?" So rather than ask someone to sit for 60 minutes a day, he found that small meditative practices, done 3 or 4 times a day for a couple minutes each time, significantly reduced stress and slowed breathing. Here's a very simple example: When you get out of bed and put your feet on the floor first thing in the morning, think of five people that you're grateful for, and think kind thoughts, and put forward good intentions. This doesn't rise to the level of deep meditation, but it can set the tone for your day.

One of the things Dr. Sood taught me, personally, was to pause before I go into a patient's room, take three deep breaths, and have kind intentions before I go in, even if it's a patient I've never met before. Dr. Sood also introduced the SMART program. SMART stands for stress management and resiliency training. It's a structured program that's scientifically proven to decrease symptoms of stress and anxiety, and increase well-being, resilience, self-regulation, mindfulness, happiness, and positive health behavior. Participants in the SMART program learn how to train their attention so that it's stronger and more focused in the present moment.

They learn to guide their thoughts based on higher principles rather than by prejudices. The program has been tested in 10 completed research studies, in and outside of Mayo Clinic, with the results showing a decrease in stress and anxiety, and an improvement in positive health behaviors.

We tried this program with new nurses here at Mayo Clinic, when they were young, and idealistic, and fresh on the job. We gave half of them a 90-minute class that taught them basic mind-body skills and how to interpret things in a positive sense—the SMART program. We followed the nurses for a year, and those trained in the SMART approach had higher job satisfaction and lower stress levels. Just being able to stop, and think, and be proactive about how you approach situations and respond to them fundamentally changes who we are.

Let's talk about one way to start the re-routing process: biofeedback. Biofeedback is a technique you can use to learn to control your body's functions, such as your heart rate. With biofeedback, you're connected to electrical sensors that help you receive information about your body. This feedback helps you focus on making subtle changes in your body, such as relaxing certain muscles, to achieve the results you want, such as reducing pain. In essence, biofeedback gives you the power to use your thoughts to control your body, often to improve a health condition or your physical performance. Biofeedback is often used as a relaxation technique. Biofeedback, sometimes called biofeedback training, is used to help manage many physical and mental health issues, including anxiety or stress, asthma, side effects from chemotherapy, chronic pain, constipation, high blood pressure, incontinence, and even irritable bowel syndrome

Although you can receive biofeedback training in physical therapy clinics, medical centers, and hospitals, more and more biofeedback devices and programs are being marketed for use at home. Some of these are hand-held portable devices while others connect to your computer. You can try different devices until you find one that works for you, or ask your doctor for advice. You might also check with your health insurance company to see what costs, if any, associated with biofeedback devices are covered.

And be aware: If a manufacturer or biofeedback practitioner claims that a biofeedback device can assess your organs for disease, or find impurities in your blood, or cure a chronic condition, or send signals into your body, do your research and check with your doctor before using it; it's probably not legitimate.

Let's talk about two of the main types of equipment used in biofeedback, and how they work. A breathing sensor monitors your breathing, helping you learn to breathe more slowly and deeply. It's also been shown to reduce blood pressure. A heart rate variability monitor shows the increases and decreases in your heart's natural cycle or rhythm. These devices measure the pulse in your fingertip or earlobe and display the time between your heartbeats. When you're stressed, the display may be jagged and spiky; when you're relaxed, the wave is smooth and consistent. By controlling your breathing, more deeply and slowly, you can change your heart rate and actually watch the wave change.

For some people, biofeedback devices like these help produce a deep state of relaxation. Other people rely on practices, such as meditation, but use biofeedback devices to assess their progress. And then other people find that devices are just distracting. You have to find what works for you. For the most part, biofeedback is widely used and accepted, and it has the potential to improve symptoms associated with many medical conditions. It has few risks, and it's practiced in many medical centers.

If biofeedback is something you're interested in, talk to your doctor. Together, you can make sure that you get proper instruction and supervision, and incorporate it as a part of a comprehensive treatment plan. Biofeedback is personally empowering and can be a good place to start if you're not ready to sign up for a yoga class, for example. Smartphone versions of biofeedback are available that you can use pretty much anywhere.

Biofeedback appeals to people because it's usually noninvasive; it may reduce or eliminate the need for medications, and it may be a treatment alternative for people who can't tolerate medications. It also helps people take charge of their health, which may mean addressing issues of control and anxiety. At Mayo Clinic, biofeedback is primarily used in our Integrative

Medicine consult service to help patients improve how they manage their stress.

Here are four main types of biofeedback techniques—the last two are the ones we use the most at Mayo Clinic for stress management. Also known as an EMG, electromyography biofeedback gives you information about the tension of your muscles to help you practice relaxation. With temperature or thermal biofeedback, sensors attached to your fingers or feet measure your skin temperature and the blood flow to your skin. Because your temperature often drops when you're under stress, a low reading may prompt you to begin relaxation techniques. In galvanic skin response training, sensors measure the activity of your sweat glands and the amount of sweat on your skin, alerting you to anxiety. And then finally, there's heart rate variability biofeedback. This type of biofeedback helps you control your heart rate in an effort to improve blood pressure, lung function, and stress and anxiety.

Here's an example of how biofeedback can help reduce stress: Researchers at Mayo Clinic studied the effects of biofeedback on a small group of nurses who care for critically ill patients. We chose this population for this study because nurses in hospitals experience a high level of stress. The study had nurses use a biofeedback-assisted, computer-guided, self-directed meditation program for 4 weeks. Over those 4 weeks, the nurses were asked to use the meditation program 4 times a week, for at least 30 minutes each time. The steps included quieting your mind, observing your thoughts, and cultivating positive emotions. This training led to improvement in stress management among the nurses who took part in the program.

You can receive biofeedback training in physical therapy clinics, medical centers, and hospitals. Typically, a biofeedback session lasts about 30–60 minutes. During a biofeedback session, a therapist will place electrical sensors on different parts of your body. These sensors monitor your body's response to stress—for example, muscle contractions during a tension headache—and then feed that information back to you through sound and visual cues. With this feedback, you start to associate your body's response—in this case, headache pain—with certain physical sensations, such as your muscles tensing. The next step is to learn how to invoke positive physical changes, such as relaxing those muscles when your body is physically or mentally stressed. Your goal is to be able to produce these responses on your own, outside the therapist's office and without the help of technology.

If you're interested in trying biofeedback to treat a muscle disorder like constipation or pelvic floor tension myalgia, the first step is to find a registered therapist. Start by asking your doctor, or another health care professional who's knowledgeable about biofeedback therapy, to recommend someone who has experience treating your condition. Otherwise, if you're interested in trying biofeedback to help manage stress, HeartMath or Relaxing Rhythms are two biofeedback tools you can try on your own.

State laws regulating biofeedback practitioners vary. Many biofeedback therapists are licensed in another area of health care, such as nursing or physical therapy, and might work under the guidance of a doctor. Some biofeedback therapists choose to become certified to show that they have extra training and experience in the practice.

When you find a potential biofeedback therapist, here are some questions to ask before starting treatment: Are you licensed, certified, or registered? If you aren't licensed, are you working under the supervision of a licensed health care professional? What is your training and experience? Do you have experience providing feedback for my condition? How many biofeedback sessions do you think I'll need? And what's the cost, and is it covered by health insurance? Can you provide a list of references?

In this lecture, we've learned a lot about some of the great ways that mind-body practices and biofeedback can be used as part of our overall health and wellness plan. Try one or both and see if they're a good fit for you. Remember, you don't have to use every approach or therapy, just the ones that make sense and fit your goals, lifestyle, and personal health needs. My hope for you as we continue exploring this exciting realm of integrative medicine is that you take away just exactly what you need to improve your health and reach your wellness goals.

Lecture 6

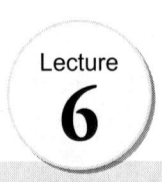

Guided Imagery, Hypnosis, and Spirituality

Aristotle and Hippocrates believed in the power of images in the brain to enliven the heart and body. Today, research shows that they were right. In this lecture, you will discover three aspects of mind-body medicine: guided imagery, hypnosis, and spirituality. Like all of the other techniques you've learned about, these methods won't change you overnight. But they can be used as part of your tool kit for mind-body health.

Guided Imagery

- Guided imagery, sometimes called visualization, is a mind-body intervention that uses the power of imagination to bring about change in your physical, emotional, or spiritual wellness. With this method of meditation, you form mental images of places or situations you find relaxing. You try to use as many senses as possible, such as smells, sights, sounds, and textures.

- Guided imagery uses the power of your imagination to guide the way your mind and body talk to each other. By imagining certain scenes in your mind, your mind can send messages to your brain that help change the way your body feels.

- From there, the message sent to your brain is passed along to the body's endocrine, immune, and autonomic nervous systems. These systems influence a wide range of bodily functions, including heart and breathing rates and blood pressure.

- Using positron-emission tomography (PET), researchers have found that the same parts of the brain are activated when people are imagining something as when they are actually experiencing it. So, if certain images bring you a feeling of peace, then incorporate them into your daily surroundings.

- Guided imagery has been shown to benefit patients by:

    o Reducing side effects from cancer treatment, including nausea, hair loss, and depression.

    o Reducing fear and anxiety prior to surgery.

    o Coping with stress.

    o Managing headaches.

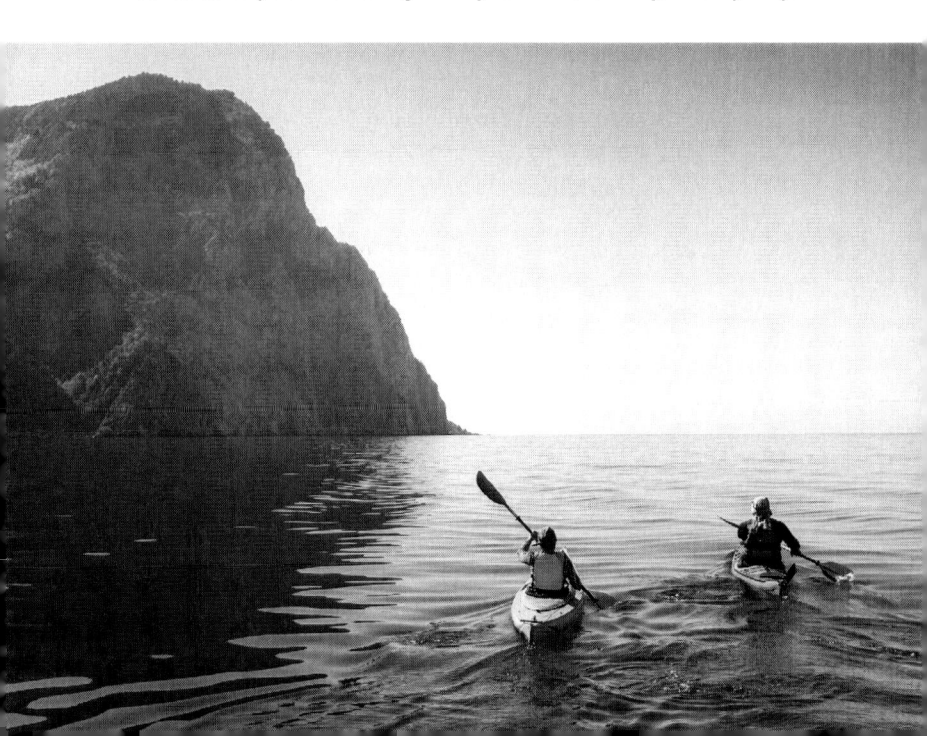

- Research has shown that when you use guided imagery to imagine a beautiful vista or a relaxing kayak ride, the image and sensations you're creating with your mind don't just stay in your mind. They affect many parts of your body, including your heart rate, blood pressure, and immune system function.

- Many people find that listening to a CD that contains guided imagery coaching to be helpful. Others choose to work one-on-one or in a small group with someone who is experienced in guided imagery.

- To make guided imagery work for you, take the following four steps.

  1. Relax. To create a desirable image, clear your mind of all chatter, worries, and distractions. Loosen tight-fitting clothing and find a comfortable, quiet place. Once you are quiet and comfortable, begin taking slow, deep breaths and release all random thoughts as you exhale.

  2. Concentrate. Focus your attention on your breathing as a way to clear your mind. If your mind wanders, acknowledge the thoughts that enter your mind and release them easily and effortlessly as you exhale. Then, refocus your attention on your breathing.

  3. Visualize. Combine a desired image with an intention, and for the next several minutes, focus on that image. You may find that your mind wanders. This may happen frequently, especially during the early stages of visualization. When it does, bring your focus back by using a slow, deep breath.

  4. Affirm. A positive affirmation coupled with the image will help create a positive message that will be stored in your brain—a message you can easily recall at a later time. Combining an image with a word or phrase may help engage both sides of your brain.

- Practicing guided imagery may feel uncomfortable or strange at first, but there's no risk. Keep an open mind and see where it takes you; you may be surprised to feel the positive effect that even just a few minutes of guided imagery can have.

Hypnotherapy

- Hypnosis, also referred to as hypnotherapy or hypnotic suggestion, is a trancelike state in which you have heightened focus and concentration. It's usually done with the help of a therapist using verbal repetition and mental images. When you're under hypnosis, you usually feel calm and relaxed and are more open to suggestions.

- There are three stages, or phases, to the process of hypnotherapy.

    1. Pre-suggestion

    2. Suggestion

    3. Post-suggestion

- The goal during pre-suggestion is to open the unconscious mind to suggestion. During the second phase, a specific thought or suggestion is presented to the subject—for example, driving over a bridge is safe, not scary. Questions may be asked and memories reviewed. Finally, in the post-suggestion stage, after returning to a normal state of consciousness, you practice the behavior that was suggested during hypnosis.

- We're not sure how hypnotherapy works in the body. Changes in skin temperature, heart rate, and immune response have been observed. Some scientists believe that hypnotherapy activates certain mind-body pathways in the nervous system.

- Hypnotherapy can be used to help you gain control over undesired behaviors or help you cope better with anxiety or pain. Although you're more open to suggestion during hypnotherapy, you don't lose control over your behavior.

- Hypnotherapy can be an effective method for coping with stress and anxiety. In particular, it can reduce stress and anxiety before a medical procedure.

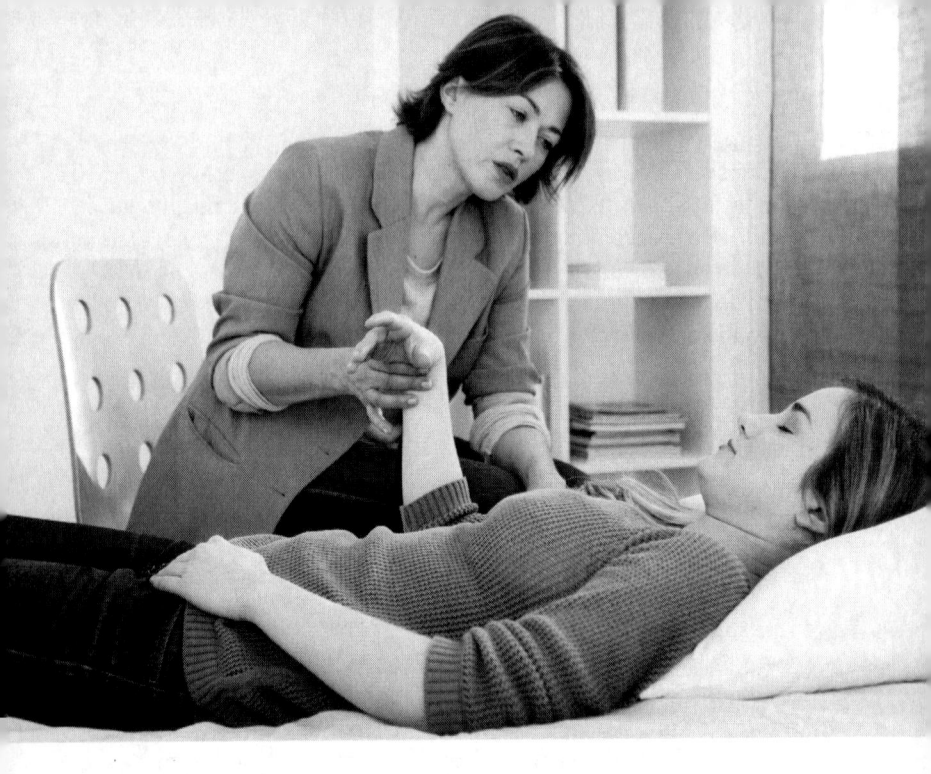

- Hypnotherapy has been studied for other conditions, including the following.

    o Pain control. Hypnotherapy may be beneficial for pain associated with cancer, irritable bowel syndrome, fibromyalgia, temporomandibular joint problems (TMJ), dental procedures, and headaches.

    o Hot flashes. Hypnotherapy may relieve symptoms of hot flashes associated with menopause.

    o Behavior change. Hypnotherapy has been used with some success in treating insomnia, bed-wetting, smoking, obesity, and phobias.

- Another interesting way that hypnotherapy is used is in weight loss. Weight loss hypnotherapy may help you shed an extra few pounds when it's part of a weight-loss plan that includes diet, exercise, and counseling. But it's difficult to say definitively if it works because there isn't enough solid scientific evidence that focuses specifically on weight loss hypnotherapy.

- Hypnotherapy that's conducted by a trained therapist or health-care professional is considered a safe complementary treatment. However, hypnotherapy may not be appropriate in people with severe mental illness.

- Adverse reactions to hypnotherapy are rare, but may include the following.

  - Headache
  - Drowsiness or dizziness
  - Anxiety or distress
  - Creation of false memories

- You don't need any special preparation to undergo hypnotherapy, but it's a good idea to wear comfortable clothing to help you relax. Also, make sure that you're well rested so that you're not inclined to fall asleep during the session.

- Be sure to carefully choose a therapist or health-care professional to perform hypnotherapy. Get a recommendation from someone you trust. Learn as much as you can about any therapist you're considering. Start by asking questions, such as the following.

  - Do you have training in a field such as psychology, medicine, or social work?
  - Are you licensed in your specialty in this state?

- How much training have you had in hypnotherapy and from what schools?

- How long have you been in practice?

- What are your fees?

- Will insurance cover your services?

• Although hypnotherapy may have the potential to help with a wide variety of conditions, it's typically used as one part of a broader treatment plan rather than as a standalone therapy. Like any other therapy, it can be very helpful to some people and not work for others. It seems to have the most success when you're highly motivated and your therapist is well trained and understands your particular problem.

Spirituality

- Spirituality has many definitions, and it's not necessarily connected to a specific belief system or even to religious worship. Instead, it arises from your connection with yourself and with others, the development of your personal value system, and your search for meaning in life.

- For many, spirituality takes the form of religious observance, prayer, meditation, or a belief in a higher power. For others, it can be found in nature, music, art, or a secular community. And some people view spirituality as experiencing a sense of peace, purpose, or connection to others or nature.

- No matter how you experience it, spirituality can help you find a sense of purpose and meaning within yourself and in your relationships with others. It can offer hope and peace during times of struggle or personal crisis. It can help lead to positive changes and improve your quality of life.

- A lot of research done on spirituality has been inconclusive, and it's been difficult to pin down exactly how it may affect people in specific ways. But researchers have found that spiritual practices may help:

  - Improve range of motion and pain in people with neck pain and restricted neck movement.

  - Decrease feelings of hopelessness in people who have idiopathic chronic pain syndrome.

  - Improve general function and reduce anxiety, depression, and symptoms of many chronic health conditions.

- Spirituality and health has become a growing field of study in medical education in the last 25 years. The field of spirituality and health is focused on the principles of service, compassion, dignity, and interconnectedness. Aiding patients' search for meaning has become more and more a focus in medical education and patient care, with an increasing number of spirituality and health courses, as well as research in this field.

- Spirituality can do a lot to help you manage your stress and benefit your overall mental health. It can help you feel a sense of purpose, connect to the world, release control, expand your support network, and lead a healthier life.

- Uncovering your spirituality may take some self-discovery. The following are some questions to ask yourself to discover what experiences and values define you.

  - What are your important relationships?

  - What do you value most in your life?

  - What people give you a sense of community?

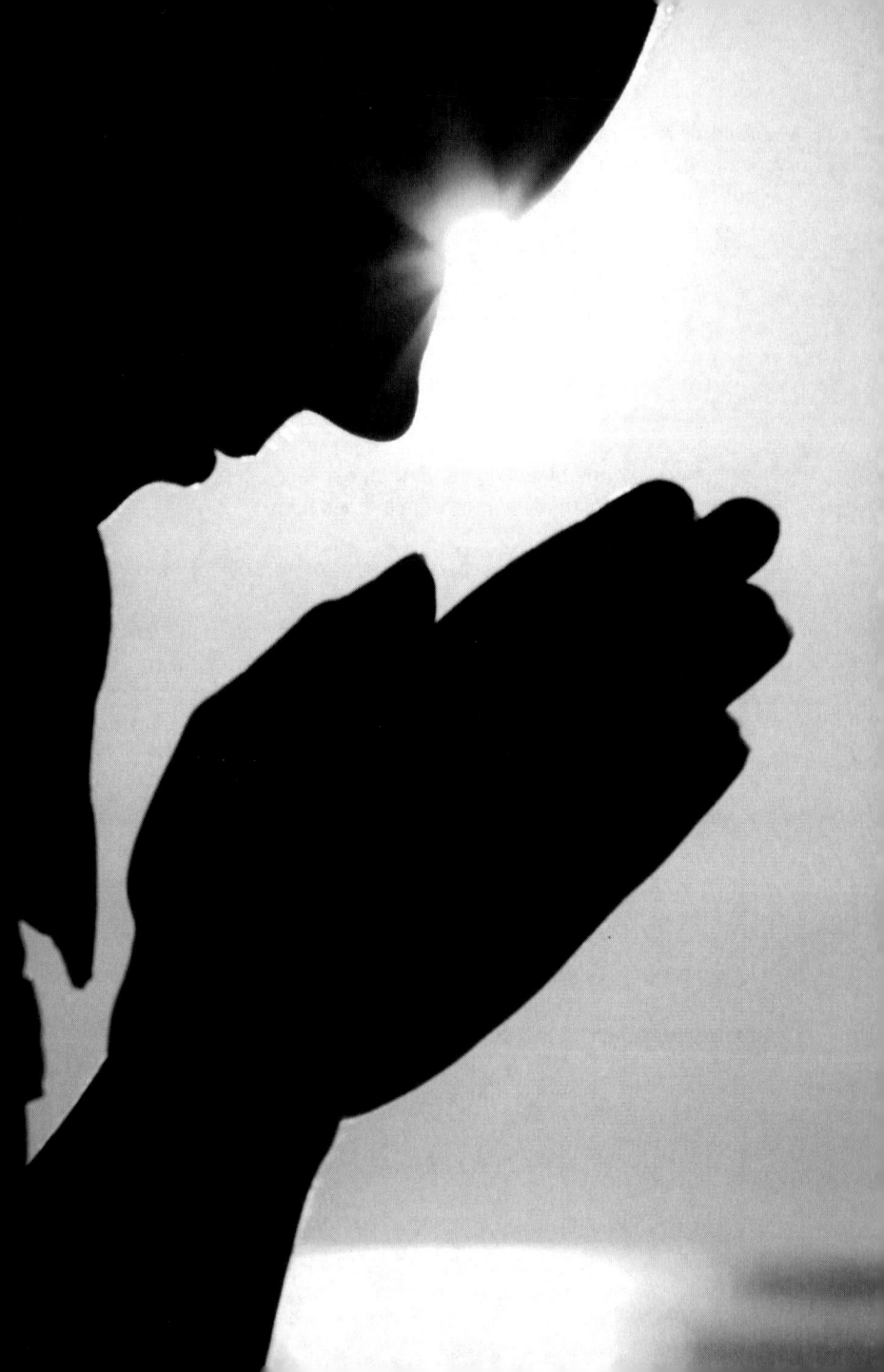

- What inspires you and gives you hope?
- What brings you joy?
- What are your proudest achievements?

- The answers to questions like these can help you identify the most important people and experiences in your life. Once you know the answers to these questions, you can focus your search for spirituality on the relationships and activities in life that have helped define you as a person and those that continue to inspire your personal growth.

- One of the best ways you can cultivate your spirituality is to foster relationships with the people who are most important to you. There are many ways you can strengthen your bond with the people you care about. The following are some ideas you can try.
  - Eat together as a family.
  - Socialize at family gatherings.
  - Be active together.
  - Take care of your friendships.

- The following activities are great ways to get in touch with your spirituality.
  - Practice prayer, meditation, and relaxation techniques to help you focus your thoughts.
  - Keep a journal to help you express your feelings and record your progress.

- - Seek out a trusted advisor or friend—someone with similar life experiences who can help you discover what's important in life.
  - Read inspirational stories or essays to help you evaluate different philosophies in life.
- Most important, be open to new experiences.
- At the same time that you're focusing inward, don't forget to cultivate the relationships in your life.
  - Work on your listening and communication skills.
  - Share your spiritual journey with loved ones.
  - Volunteer within your community.
  - See the good in people and yourself.

Suggested Reading

Dasse, et al, "Hypnotizability, Not Suggestion, Influences False Memory Development."

Foji, et al, "The Study of the Effect of Guided Imagery."

Gonzales, et al, "Effects of Guided Imagery on Postoperative Outcomes."

Halpin, et al, "Guided Imagery in Cardiac Surgery."

Kwekkeboom, et al, "Patients' Perceptions of the Effectiveness of Guided Imagery."

Lang, "Americans' Circle of Confidantes Has Shrunk to Two People."

Natural Medicines Research Collaboration, "Spiritual Healing."

Lecture 6 Transcript

Guided Imagery, Hypnosis, and Spirituality

Aristotle and Hippocrates believed in the power of images in the brain to enliven the heart and body. Today, research shows they were right. In this lecture, we're going to touch on three aspects of mind-body medicine: guided imagery, hypnosis, and spirituality and prayer.

At Mayo Clinic, I have the opportunity on a daily basis to see guided imagery help patients use the full range of the body's healing capacity. Guided imagery is more than listening to relaxing sounds; it's a mind-body intervention that uses the power of imagination to bring about change in your physical, emotional, or spiritual wellness. Sometimes called guided imagery or visualization, with this method of meditation you form mental images of places or situations you find relaxing.

You try to use as many senses as possible, such as smells, sights, sounds, and textures. Guided imagery uses the power of your imagination to guide the way your mind and body talk to each other. By imagining certain scenes in your mind, your mind can send messages to your brain that can help change the way your body feels. For example, you may feel more relaxed or feel less pain. From there, the message sent to your brain is passed along to the body's endocrine, immune, and autonomic nervous systems. These systems influence a wide range of bodily functions, including heart and breathing rates and blood pressure.

Using positron-emission tomography, known as a PET scan, researchers have found that the same parts of the brain are activated when people are imagining something as when they are actually experiencing it. For example, when someone imagines a serene image, the optic cortex—the part of the brain that processes visual images—is activated in the same way as when the person is actually seeing the beautiful vista. So if having a nature scene on your computer or hanging on your wall relaxes or soothes, go for it. If certain images bring you a feeling of peace, then by all means, incorporate them into your daily surroundings.

Guided imagery has been shown to benefit patients by: Reducing side effects from cancer treatment, including nausea, hair loss, and depression. Reducing fear and anxiety prior to surgery—studies have actually shown that surgery patients who participated in two to four guided imagery sessions needed less pain medication and left the hospital more quickly than those who hadn't used imagery. Coping with stress. Managing headaches—studies have shown that guided imagery may help reduce the frequency of migraine headaches as effectively as taking preventive medications.

A study by the American Association of Nurse Anesthetists evaluated the effects of guided imagery on post-operative outcomes in patients undergoing same-day surgery. In the study, some patients listened to a CD with a guided imagery demonstration, and the others simply had privacy. The patients who listened to the CD reported significantly lower levels of anxiety and significantly less pain after surgery, and they were even discharged from the hospital a little bit earlier.

In another study, guided imagery was used on patients undergoing cardiac surgery. Researchers wanted to see if a guided imagery program could reduce anxiety, pain, and the length of stay at a decreased cost to the consumer while still maintaining a high level of patient satisfaction. In terms of their overall care and the treatment they received, there were no statistically significant differences between patients in the guided imagery group and those not in the group. But patients who used guided imagery before and after surgery reported higher satisfaction and less anxiety—a 41% improvement—compared to those who didn't use guided imagery.

Guided imagery has even used to help improved a person's golf swing or a piano performance. For example, in a study involving 62 high school students, participants took an 8-week program that taught them cognitive skills they could use to help improve their music performance and reduce their performance anxiety. Mental rehearsal, including imagining and visualizing the performance, helped the students feel less anxious when it came time for their actual performances.

All of the research that I've mentioned leads to one important point: When you use guided imagery to imagine a beautiful vista or taking a relaxing kayak ride, the images and sensations you're creating with your mind don't just stay in your mind. They affect many parts of your body, including your heart rate, blood pressure, even how your immune system functions.

Many people find listening to a CD that contains guided imagery coaching to be helpful. Others choose to work one-on-one or in a small group with someone who's experienced in guided imagery. To make guided imagery work for you, take these four steps:

Step one, relax. To create a desirable image, clear your mind of all chatter, worries, and distractions. Loosen tight-fitting clothing; find a comfortable, quiet place. Once you are quiet and comfortable, begin taking slow, deep breaths and release all random thoughts as you exhale.

Step number two, concentrate. Focus your attention on your breathing as a way to clear your mind. If your mind wanders, acknowledge the thoughts that enter your mind and release them easily and effortlessly as you exhale. Then, refocus your attention on your breathing.

Step three, visualize. Now, combine a desired image with an intention, and for the next several minutes, focus on that image. For example, picture a good friend that you've lost touch with and make an intention to reconnect with that person. You may find that your mind wanders. This may happen frequently, especially during the early stages of visualization. When it does, bring your focus back by using a slow, deep breath.

Step four, affirm. A positive affirmation, coupled with the image, will help to create a positive message that will be stored in your brain; a message you can easily recall at a later time. Combining an image with a word or phrase may help to engage both sides of your brain.

Practicing guided imagery may feel uncomfortable or strange at first, but there's no risk here. Keep an open mind and see where it takes you—you may be surprised to feel the positive effect that even just a few minutes of guided imagery can have.

When it comes to the use of complementary methods for treatment and prevention, cancer is an area of significant research and practice. Guided imagery is an established intervention in integrative oncology. In one study, patients who were undergoing radiation therapy for breast cancer participated in guided imagery and were monitored via biofeedback—which we discussed in an earlier lecture. Researchers could see how guided imagery affected the patients' blood pressure, breathing rate, pulse rate, and skin temperature. They found that a 30-minute guided imagery session was helpful for the patients—their skin temperature increased, indicating better blood flow; and their breathing rates, blood pressure, and pulse were all reduced.

In another cancer-related study, this time from the University of Wisconsin-Madison School of Nursing, researchers took a look at how guided imagery affected pain in 26 cancer patients, ranging in age from 18–72 years. More than half the patients said that guided imagery helped relieve their pain. Those who felt that guided imagery was helpful said that the exercise helped distract them from their pain. Some said that the voice leading the exercise was soothing; for others, the imagery involved in the exercise got them to focus their concentration on something other than the pain. Still others felt that the most useful part of guided imagery was simply the relaxation it brought. The benefits of guided imagery don't end with cancer; it's been explored for many other medical conditions, including arthritis and other rheumatic diseases, to treat symptoms of heart failure before and after heart surgery, and during pregnancy.

Most of us have heard the word mesmerize. It comes from the name of a German doctor, Franz Anton Mesmer, who is considered to be one of the founders of modern Western hypnotherapy. Mesmer believed that illness was caused by an imbalance of magnetic fluids in the body, and that this imbalance could be corrected by transferring the hypnotist's own magnetism to the individual. In the late 1700s, Mesmer used this technique to help heal many serious diseases, including pain and severe sensory disabilities.

Forms of hypnosis, trance, and altered states of consciousness have been used by many cultures and civilizations throughout history. Modern science understands hypnosis—also referred to as hypnotherapy, or hypnotic suggestion—to be a trance-like state in which you have heightened focus and concentration. It's usually done with the help of a therapist using verbal repetition and mental images. When you're under hypnosis, you usually feel calm and relaxed and are more open to suggestions. There are three stages or phases to the process of hypnotherapy: pre-suggestion, suggestion, post-suggestion.

The goal during pre-suggestion is to open the unconscious mind to suggestion. During the second phase, a specific thought or suggestion is presented to the subject—you don't want to smoke; or driving over a bridge is safe, not scary. Questions may be asked and memories reviewed. Finally, in the post-suggestion stage, after returning to a normal state of consciousness, you practice the behavior that was suggested during hypnosis. We're not sure how hypnotherapy works in the body. Changes in skin temperature, heart rate, and immune response have been observed. Some scientists believe that hypnotherapy activates certain mind-body pathways in the nervous system.

While hypnotherapy is often portrayed humorously on TV and in movies, it can be an effective treatment for some people. Research shows that certain individuals connect with hypnotherapy more than others do. Hypnotherapy can be used to help you gain control over undesired behaviors, or to help you cope better with anxiety or pain. It's important to know that although you're more open to suggestion during hypnotherapy, you don't lose control over your behavior. Hypnotherapy can be an effective method for coping with stress and anxiety. In particular, it can reduce stress and anxiety before a medical procedure, such as a breast biopsy.

Hypnotherapy has been studied for other conditions, including pain control. Hypnotherapy may be beneficial for pain associated with cancer, irritable bowel syndrome, fibromyalgia, temporomandibular joint problems—

also known as TMJ—dental procedures, and headaches. Hot flashes. Hypnotherapy may relieve symptoms of hot flashes associated with menopause. Behavior change. Hypnotherapy has been used with some success in treating insomnia, bed-wetting, smoking, obesity, and phobias.

Another interesting way that hypnotherapy is used is in weight loss. Weight-loss hypnotherapy may help you shed an extra few pounds when it's part of a weight-loss program that includes diet, exercise, and counseling. But it's hard to say definitively if it works because there isn't enough solid scientific evidence that focuses specifically on weight-loss hypnotherapy. A few studies have evaluated the use of weight-loss hypnotherapy. Most studies show only slight weight loss, with an average loss of about 6 pounds. But the quality of some of these studies has been questioned, making it hard to determine the true effectiveness of weight-loss hypnotherapy. Weight loss is usually best achieved with diet and exercise. If you've tried diet and exercise but are still struggling to meet your weight-loss goal, talk to your health care provider about other options or lifestyle changes that you can make. Don't rely on weight-loss hypnotherapy alone because it's unlikely to lead to significant weight loss.

Hypnotherapy that's conducted by a trained therapist or health care professional is considered a safe, complementary treatment. However, hypnotherapy may not be appropriate in people with severe mental illness.

Adverse reactions to hypnotherapy are rare, but may include: headache, drowsiness or dizziness, anxiety or distress, and even creation of false memories.

Use special caution before using hypnotherapy for age regression, to help you relive earlier events in your life. This practice remains controversial and has limited scientific evidence to support its use. It may cause strong emotions, and can alter your memories or lead to creation of false memories. In a 2015 study, Baylor University researchers found that how susceptible people are to suggestion under hypnosis plays a significant role in whether or not hypnotherapy will lead to the creation of false memories. More study needs to be done in this area to understand exactly what and how much of a role susceptibility to hypnotherapy plays in the creation of false memories, but it is a possible drawback of hypnotherapy to be aware of. You don't need any special preparation to undergo hypnotherapy, but it's a good idea to wear comfortable clothing to help you relax. Also, make sure that you're well rested so that you're not inclined to fall asleep during the session.

Be sure you carefully choose a therapist or health care professional to perform hypnotherapy. Get a recommendation from someone you trust. Learn as much as you can about any therapist you're considering. Start by asking questions, such as: Do you have training in a field such as psychology, medicine, or social work? Are you licensed in your specialty in this state? How much training have you had in hypnotherapy, and from what schools? How long have you been in practice? What are your fees? And will insurance cover your services?

During a hypnotherapy session, the therapist will explain the process of hypnosis and review what you hope to accomplish. Then the therapist will typically talk in a gentle, soothing tone and describe images that create a sense of relaxation, security, and well-being. When you're in a receptive state, the therapist will suggest ways for you to achieve your goals, such as reducing pain or eliminating cravings to smoke. The therapist also may help you visualize vivid, meaningful mental images of yourself accomplishing your goals. When the session is over, either you're able to bring yourself out of hypnosis, or your therapist helps you end your trance-like state.

Contrary to how hypnotherapy is sometimes portrayed in movies or on television, you don't lose control over your behavior while under hypnotherapy. Also, you generally remain aware of, and remember, what happens under hypnosis. You may eventually be able to practice self-hypnosis, in which you induce a state of hypnosis yourself. You can use this skill as needed—for instance, after a chemotherapy session.

Although hypnotherapy may have the potential to help with a wide variety of conditions, it's not a magic bullet. It's typically used as one part of a broader treatment plan rather than as a stand-alone therapy. Like any other therapy, it can be very helpful to some people and not work with others. It seems to have the most success when you're highly motivated, and your therapist is well trained and understands your particular problem.

Biofeedback, hypnosis, and guided imagery are three very specific practices and therapies to address the mind-body connection. But at the very beginning of this course, you may remember that we also discussed very tangible strategies that can improve your well-being, mind, body, and soul. Those strategies were exercising more, eating healthy foods, managing stress, and staying connected to friends and family.

Spirituality is another one of those tangible strategies—another tool in the mind-body health kit—but it's not as simple as eating whole grains or getting 150 minutes of physical activity each week. Spirituality means something different to everyone. Spirituality has many definitions, and it's not necessarily connected to a specific belief system or even to religious worship. Instead, it arises from your connection with yourself and with others, the development of your personal value system, and your search for meaning in life.

For many, spirituality takes the form of religious observance, prayer, meditation, or a belief in a higher power. For others, it can be found in nature, music, art, or a secular community. And some people view spirituality as experiencing a sense of peace, purpose, or connections to others or nature. No matter how you experience it, spirituality can help you find a sense of purpose and meaning within yourself, and in your relationship with others. It can offer hope and peace during times of struggle or personal crisis. It can help lead to positive changes and improve your quality of life.

A lot of research done on spirituality has been inconclusive, and it's been hard to pin down exactly how it may affect people in specific ways. But researchers have found that spiritual practices may help improve range of motion and pain with people with neck pain and restricted neck movement; decrease feelings of hopelessness in people who have idiopathic chronic pain syndrome; improve general function and reduce anxiety, depression, and symptoms of many chronic health conditions

In North America, as many as 43% of people use prayer to improve their health. Spirituality and health have become a growing field of study in medical education in the last 25 years. A field of study called spirituality and health is focused on the principles of service, compassion, dignity, and interconnectedness. Aiding patients' search for meaning has become more and more of a focus in medical education and patient care, with an increasing number of spirituality and health courses, as well as research in this field.

Kate Piderman, a chaplain at Mayo Clinic Hospice and coordinator of research for Chaplain Services at Mayo Clinic, has seen spirituality improve many people's lives over the years, and has watched as spirituality has helped people maintain a positive attitude during a time of serious medical illness. She explains spirituality well; I'll quote her here: She says that,

> Spirituality is an opportunity to experience life at the deepest level. In its best sense—she says—spirituality offers beliefs, practices, and relationships that form the way you relate to yourself and others. It gives you a way to approach each day with wonder and gratitude, grace and generosity, meaning and purpose. Spirituality helps you see the blessings in each day and helps motivate you to add to the goodness of all.

You probably practice spirituality every day without even realizing it. Ask yourself these questions: Have you connected with others, such as friends, family, or a group that gathers for a spiritual purpose? Have you helped someone in need? Have you been able to look at the bigger picture in life, especially during times of stress? Do you enjoy spending time in nature? Have you experienced God or a higher power at work in your life? Do you take part in activities such as prayer, meditation, deep breathing, expressing gratitude, silent observation, or experiencing art? Do you look for and do things that give your life meaning and purpose, such as the work you do or something that helps you feel connected to something larger than yourself? You may be surprised to know that each and every one of these activities can be seen as a spiritual activity.

Spirituality can do a lot to help you manage your stress and benefit your overall mental health. Spirituality can help you feel a sense of purpose. Cultivating your spirituality may help uncover what's most meaningful in your life. By clarifying what's most important, you can focus less on the unimportant things and eliminate stress.

It can help you connect to the world. The more you feel you have a purpose in the world, the less solitary you feel—even when you're alone. This can lead to a valuable inner peace during difficult times. A 2011 Cornell University study found that Americans have become increasingly isolated. Most people had only two people they felt close to, and the number of people who felt they didn't have a close relationship with anyone tripled between 1985 and 2004. Spirituality helps you release control. When you feel part of a greater whole, you realize that you aren't responsible for everything that happens in life. You can share the burden of tough times, as well as the joys of life's blessings, with those around you.

Spirituality can also help you expand your support network. Whether you find spirituality in a church, mosque or synagogue, in your family, or in nature walks with a friend, this sharing of spiritual expression can help build relationships. And finally, spirituality can help you lead a healthier life. People who consider themselves spiritual appear to be better able to cope with stress, and heal from illness or addiction faster.

Uncovering your spirituality may take some self-discovery. Here are some questions to ask yourself to discover what experiences and values define you: What are your important relationships? What do you value most in your life? What people give you a sense of community? What inspires you and gives you hope? What brings you joy? What are your proudest achievements?

The answers to questions like these can help you identify the most important people and experiences in your life. Once you know the answers to these questions, you can focus your search for spirituality on the relationships and activities in life that have helped define you as a person, and those that continue to inspire your personal growth. We've lost a lot of the spiritual connection in our lives. When I ask people about their community, their relationships, their spirituality, they often don't have an answer.

For the younger generation, a lot of this is due to technology. Technology has helped us in many ways, but it's also distanced us as a community. I see younger people having trouble looking people in the eye, or having a conversation, or having an emotional connection because so much of how they communicate is done online. There's also less of a focus on family interaction and communication. We're so busy running around, and everyone has a separate schedule. We've lost that family dinner where we sit and talk about our day and about what's going on in our family's and friends' lives. We've become very self-focused.

Part of this started in the 1960s when the younger generation moved away from religion. Back then, religion was a foundation of community; you went to church every week, and everyone knew each other, and you also learned the basic values of taking care of each other. When someone was sick, people helped with food, or chores, or babysitting. Now where do you go to find that example? Of course, some families volunteer, and many people still belong to churches or synagogues; but we've gotten away from having that common connection to each other, as well as that deeper faith. That connection—to ourselves and to others—is how a sense of spirituality begins, and how it ultimately leads to finding a sense of purpose in life.

With all of this in mind, one of the best ways you can cultivate your spirituality is to foster relationships with the people who are most important to you. There are a lot of ways you can strengthen your bond with the people you care about. I like to follow Dr. Sood's suggestion to greet your family members when you walk in the door as if you've been away for 3 months. Try to just appreciate them for who they are, don't try to correct or improve them—for at least 5 minutes anyway.

Here are some more ideas you can try: Eat together as a family. Family meals can help you influence children's behavior and development. Studies show that adolescents who share family meals have healthier eating habits and body weight, do better in school, have a better psychological well-being, and are less likely to get into drugs and alcohol, or other trouble.

Socialize at family gatherings. Planning and preparing healthy meals is important, but so is taking the time to enjoy what you eat and visit with family and friends at family gatherings.

Be active together. Go to community events or races, volunteer and give back to others, go for a walk, or meet up at a park—whatever gets you out doing something together. This gives you the chance to be active, but it can also give you a chance to have experiences together and build good memories as a family.

Take care of your friendships. Maintaining healthy relationships requires a little give and take. Try to respect your friends' boundaries, don't compete, and don't complain too much—these are all things that can hurt friendships. Take a genuine interest in what's going on in your friends' lives, and don't judge them. Give your family and friends space to change, grow, and make mistakes; and keep confidential any personal information that they share. Investing time in making friends and strengthening your friendships can pay off in better health.

At Mayo Clinic, we have a meditation room that offers a quiet, peaceful environment for staff, patients, and family members to rest, replenish, and rejuvenate. With soft lighting, gentle music, and the soothing sound of a water fountain, the meditation room provides a transition to tranquility and contemplation. The meditation room offers the opportunity to take a moment for quiet sitting and centering; listen to gentle healing music and sounds of water falling; meditate; offer prayers; read for comfort or enjoyment; listen to guided imagery or relaxation tapes; talk to a friend, counselor, spiritual advisor; write in a journal.

All of these activities are great ways to get in touch with your own spirituality. But you don't have to have access to Mayo Clinic's meditation room to become more spiritual; there are many other things you can do. If you aren't sure how to start, think back to some of the techniques I mentioned earlier in this lecture. Practice prayer, meditation, and relaxation techniques to help you focus your thoughts. Keep a journal to help you express your feelings and record your progress. Seek out a trusted advisor or friend—someone with similar life experiences who can help you discover what's important in life. Read inspirational stories or essays to help you evaluate different philosophies in life. Most important, be open to new experiences. You aren't going to turn into the Dalai Lama in a single day. If your spirituality is more secular, you might consider expanding your horizons with new experiences in the arts.

At the same time that you're focusing inward, don't forget to cultivate the relationships in your life. Work on your listening and communication skills. Maybe listen to a lecture on active listening and practice it in a conversation with a friend. How does it change the conversation? How do you feel afterward? Share your spiritual journey with loved ones. Volunteer within your community. See the good in people and yourself. Notice when someone does something kind, whether it's letting someone go ahead in line, or a dental assistant giving your shoulder a squeeze if you're nervous.

Like everything else we've discussed, these changes won't happen overnight. If you're used to flipping off other drivers on the road or yelling at the walls when you've lost your keys, again, it's going to take time to create those calmer pathways and make connections to new people. Don't rush it and take a second to notice when you do react in a different, more positive way. It all builds up in the long run.

Lecture 7

Practicing Meditation

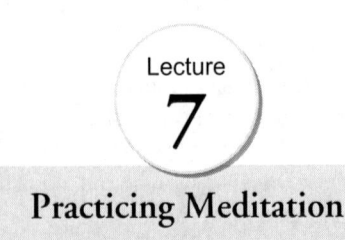

Many meditation techniques have roots in Eastern religious or spiritual traditions, and some people consider praying a form of meditation. But like many of the mind-body practices you've encountered in this course, there's no one right way to meditate. No matter how you meditate, the goal is the same: to focus your attention. As you will learn in this lecture, the idea behind meditation is to suspend the stream of thoughts that normally occupies your conscious mind, leading to a state of physical relaxation, mental calmness, and psychological balance.

Understanding Meditation

- Amit Sood, M.D., the head of Mayo Clinic's Mind-Body Initiative, says that it's common for people to struggle when they first start a meditation practice. That's because American life tends to be complex and busy.

- One of the biggest challenges is addressing the constant state of anxiety that Americans have. People worry that if they're still and quiet instead of constantly thinking about which undone task they have to do next, they will make a mistake and one of those tasks will not get done. Being busy all of the time often makes people feel like they're handling life much better; slowing down or stopping feels uncomfortable.

- The second challenge is learning to be mentally still. Dr. Sood says that the brain wanders on purpose on an evolutionary level. If we were cavemen and were sitting still in the middle of a forest with our eyes closed, not paying attention to what's around us, that might be problematic—and even life-threatening.

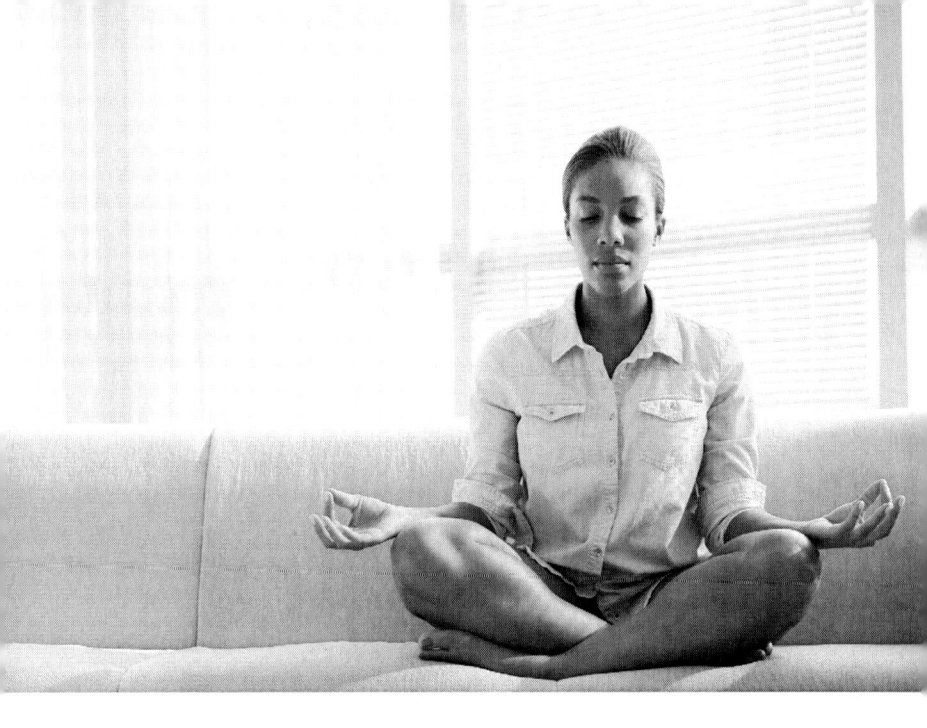

- So, one of the first things we have to accept is that our minds are going to wander. In fact, the mind spends most of the day wandering. Trying to focus this wandering mind goes against human nature.

- Being physically still—actually sitting still—is a similar challenge. You might feel an itch or pain in your back, or you might get fidgety. That's all okay. It's okay, too, to meditate in the way that works best for you.

- Sometimes patients are worried that if they try to sit still and meditate, they'll fail. For these individuals, meditation is one more thing they feel bad about not doing—one of the undone tasks taking up space in their minds. These individuals should try different practices until they find one that works for them.

- Dr. Sood says that the final challenge in learning to meditate is laziness. Meditation, like everything else, is a discipline. You have to commit time to it, and like any new habit or behavior, it may require a little extra effort at first.

- Some people have unrealistic expectations about how meditation will affect their lives. They may expect an out-of-body experience with lights and sounds or that their anger will suddenly disappear. For most people, these things don't usually happen during meditation.

- You might discover that as soon as you let yourself relax when meditating, you fall asleep. If this is a problem for you, you could try doing meditation earlier in the day or use a sitting, rather than a lying-down, posture. True meditation should be at the cusp of relaxation—when you're still awake and alert.

- When you meditate, you want to clear away the information overload that builds up every day and contributes to your stress.

- Emotional benefits of meditation can include:

    o   Gaining a new perspective on stressful situations.

    o   Building skills to manage your stress.

    o   Increasing self-awareness.

    o   Being able to focus on the present moment.

    o   Reducing negative emotions.

    o   Improving your memory and concentration.

    o   Helping you stick to a physical activity program.

Four Steps to Starting Meditation

1. **Find a quiet place.** Try to find a quiet place with few distractions. The more often you practice meditation, the easier it will be for you to meditate, even with traffic blaring around you.
2. **Choose your posture.** Is sitting against a wall comfortable for you? What about sitting on a cushion or in a favorite chair? Are you most comfortable lying down? These are all fine postures.
3. **Focus your attention.** Maybe you want to choose a word to repeat, or you can light a candle and focus on the flame.
4. **Keep an open mind.** Let distractions come and go without engaging them. If they happen, let them go and bring your attention back to the focus.

- Meditation might also be useful if you have a medical condition, especially one that may be worsened by stress.

- Some research suggests that meditation can help people manage symptoms of conditions such as anxiety disorders, asthma, cancer, depression, heart disease, high blood pressure, pain, and sleep problems.

- Researchers at Harvard found that participating in an eight-week mindfulness meditation program appears to make measurable changes in the parts of the brain associated with memory, sense of self, empathy, and stress. At UCLA, researchers found that the brains of long-term meditators were better preserved than the brains of non-meditators as they aged.

- In some circumstances, we know that meditation helps, but we're not sure why. A meta-analysis at Johns Hopkins University focused on the relationship between mindfulness meditation and its ability to reduce symptoms of depression, anxiety, and pain. Researchers found that among people with depression, meditation produced a response similar to that of antidepressants. This is an interesting finding, and one day, meditation might become part of a care plan for depression.

How Meditation Works

- Practicing meditation has been shown to produce physical changes, such as in the body's fight-or-flight response. The system responsible for this response is called the autonomic nervous system, sometimes called the involuntary nervous system, which regulates many activities, including your heartbeat, blood pressure, perspiration, breathing rate, body temperature, the production of body fluids, and digestion.

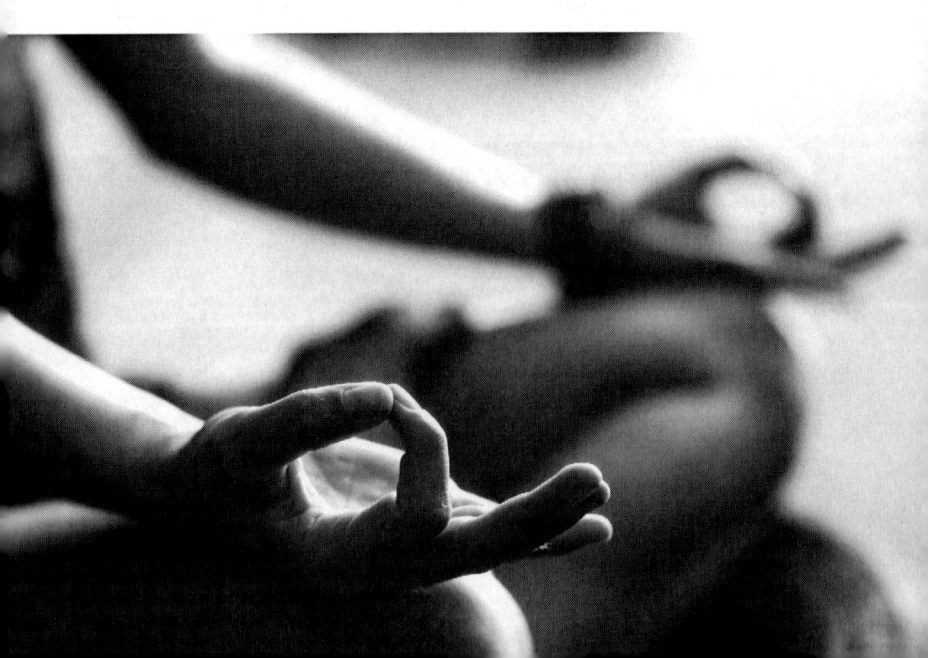

- The autonomic nervous system is divided into the sympathetic nervous system and the parasympathetic nervous system. The sympathetic nervous system helps mobilize the body into action—the fight-or-flight response. The parasympathetic nervous system, or the so-called rest-and-digest system, slows your heartbeat, allowing your blood vessels to dilate and improving blood flow. Research is focusing on how meditation may reduce the activity of the sympathetic nervous system and increase that of the parasympathetic system.

- Research has also shown that meditation can be an effective way to slow our brain waves—slow down all of the traffic in our head—so that the body and mind can work in tandem. As each breath begins to lengthen, the brain waves begin to slow.

- You can take the first step toward starting a meditation program simply by setting aside time each day to incorporate some quiet reflection in your life, quieting your mind a little and focusing on just one thing.

- If one kind of meditation doesn't work for you, try something else that may be more your speed—tai chi or yoga or going for a quiet walk. Whatever you can do to try to quiet your mind and let the thoughts flow by, that's what works for you.

- For some people, it's a struggle to keep very quiet, and they get frustrated and think they're not doing it right. Maybe sitting for 15 minutes in silence is a long-range goal, and that's okay. What's important is to start somewhere, no matter where it is, doing something that works for you.

- If sitting in silence for 15 minutes doesn't work for you right now, maybe a practice that makes more sense for you is to focus on compassionate thoughts or kind intentions. In these cases, you're not sitting down to meditate; instead, you're being mindful toward the people you meet. That's meditation, too.

Styles of Meditation
- If you're thinking about starting a meditation practice, the following are a few options to start with.

    o Analytical meditation is when you try to comprehend the deeper meaning of an object you're focusing on. In analytical meditation, you might focus your attention on a scriptural passage or a concept—maybe how precious human life is. Through this type of meditation, the goal is to focus on feeling empathy and compassion toward yourself and toward others.

- Breath meditation involves focusing on your breathing, consciously observing every inhalation and exhalation and the rising and falling of the chest. Breathing that is deep, slow, and smooth and that comes from your diaphragm is maintained in this practice. The purpose is to slow your breathing, take in more oxygen, and reduce the use of shoulder, neck, and upper chest muscles while breathing so that you breathe more efficiently.

- Mindfulness meditation is based on the concept of having an increased awareness and acceptance of the present moment. One mindfulness meditation exercise is to bring all your attention to the sensation and flow of air moving in and out of your body. The goal is to focus on what you're experiencing in the present moment without reacting to it or making any judgments about it.

- Body scanning means that you focus attention on different parts of your body. Through body scanning, you become aware of your body's various sensations—whether that's pain, tension, warmth, or relaxation. You can combine body scanning with breathing exercises and imagine breathing heat or relaxation into and out of different parts of your body.

- Transcendental meditation teaches you to focus on a mantra—a sound, word, or phrase—that you repeat over and over, either out loud or to yourself. The goal is to keep distracting thoughts out of your conscious awareness. You can create your own mantra, whether it's religious or secular. Whatever mantra you choose, it should hold your attention on a single thought or sensation that brings you a sense of comfort. This type of training is offered for a fee (for more information, visit www.tm.org/learn-tm).

Types of Meditation

- **Walking meditation**
  With walking meditation, called *kinhin* in the Zen tradition, you focus on the subtle movements used to stand and walk. You can use this technique anywhere you're walking, such as in a tranquil forest, on a city sidewalk, or at the mall.

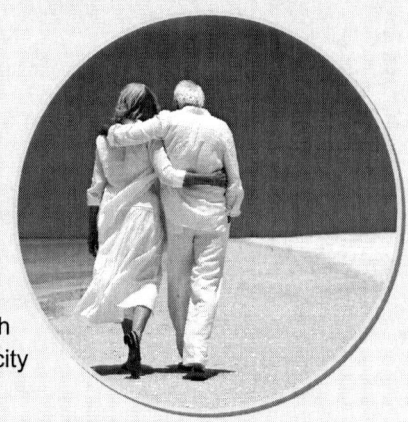

  When you use this method, slow down your pace so that you can focus on each movement of your legs or feet. Don't focus on a particular destination. Concentrate on your legs and feet, repeating action words in your mind, such as "lifting," "moving," and "placing," as you lift each foot. Move your leg forward and place your foot on the ground.

- **Guided meditation**
  Similar to guided imagery, or visualization, techniques, with guided meditation, you form mental images of places or situations you find relaxing. Try to use as many senses as possible, such as smells, sights, sounds, and textures. You may be led through this process in a class by a guide or teacher, or you may prefer to use guided imagery programs on your own at home.

- **Focus your love and gratitude**
  In this type of meditation, you focus your attention on a sacred object or being, weaving feelings of love, compassion, and gratitude into your thoughts. You can also close your eyes and use your imagination or gaze at representations of the object.

Suggested Reading

Creagan, et al, "Animal-Assisted Therapy at Mayo Clinic."

Cutshall, et al, "A Decade of Offering a Healing Enhancement Program."

Cutshall, et al, "Creation of a Healing Enhancement Program."

Goyal, et al, "Meditation Programs for Psychological Stress and Wellbeing."

Holzel, et al, "Mindfulness Practice Leads to Increases in Regional Brain Gray Matter."

Luders, Eileen, et al, "Forever Young(er)."

Lecture 7 Transcript

Practicing Meditation

The word meditation has become part of our everyday vocabulary. We hear people talking about meditating on television, sports figures say they meditate as part of their exercise routine, and even some elementary schools are incorporating meditation into their curriculums.

But really, the term meditation refers to a group of techniques. Many meditation techniques have roots in Eastern religious or spiritual traditions, and some people consider praying a form of meditation. But like a lot of the mind-body practices we've discussed, there's no one right way to meditate.

No matter how you meditate, the goal is really the same—to focus your attention. Maybe your focus is on your breathing, as you inhale and exhale, or on a specific word that you're repeating. Or maybe you meditate by taking a moment of gratitude before you sit down at your desk.

The idea behind meditation is to suspend the stream of thoughts that normally occupies your conscious mind. This leads to a state of physical relaxation, mental calmness, and psychological balance. Practicing meditation can change how you relate to the flow of your emotions and thoughts, and it may help you control how you respond to a challenging situation. For example, if you're claustrophobic and you know you're going to have an MRI, meditating and focusing on your breathing as you inhale and exhale may help you feel less anxious and get through the exam. Or maybe public speaking makes you nervous, so you take five deep breaths before giving a big presentation to help you slow down, relax, and focus.

Anyone can practice meditation. It's simple and inexpensive, and you don't need any special equipment to do it. You can practice meditation wherever you are—whether you're out for a walk, riding the bus, waiting at the doctor's office, or even in the middle of a difficult business meeting. Meditation has been practiced for thousands of years. It originally was meant to help deepen understanding of the sacred and mystical forces of life.

There are a lot of misconceptions about meditation, particularly for older people who grew up with The Beatles. They may think meditating means having to go to India and find a guru and live in a cave or that you have to be some sort of mystic or that it's tied to religion. But this isn't the only reason that people struggle with just the idea of meditation.

Dr. Amit Sood, whom I've mentioned in earlier lectures—he chairs the Mayo Clinic Mind-Body Initiative in Mayo Clinic's Complementary and Integrative Medicine Program. Dr. Sood says it's common for people to struggle when they first start a meditation practice. That's because American life tends to be complex and busy, and people have a lot going on—with something like 150 undone tasks all at the same time.

One of the biggest challenges is addressing that constant state of anxiety that Americans have. People worry that if they sit still and are quiet instead of constantly thinking about what they have to do next, one of those balls will drop. Being busy all of the time often makes people feel like they're handling life a lot better. Slowing down or stopping feels uncomfortable.

The second challenge is learning to be mentally still. Dr. Sood says the brain wanders on purpose on an evolutionary level. If we were cavemen, and we were sitting still in the middle of a forest with our eyes closed not paying attention to what's around us—that might be problematic and even life-threatening.

So one of the first things we have to accept is that our minds are going to wander. In fact, the mind spends most of the day wandering. Trying to focus this wandering goes against human nature. Being physically still— actually sitting still—is a similar challenge. You might feel an itch, your back may hurt, your muscles may cramp, or you may get fidgety. That's all okay. With all of this said, remember, too, that it's okay to meditate in the way that works best for you. Not everyone who meditates sits on the floor in the shape of a pretzel.

Sometimes patients tell me they're worried that if they try to sit still and meditate, they'll fail. For these individuals, meditation was one more thing they felt bad about not doing—one of those 150 undone tasks taking up space in their minds that I mentioned earlier. I encourage these individuals to try different practices until they find one that works for them.

Dr. Sood says the final challenge in learning to meditate is laziness. Meditation, like everything else, is a discipline. You have to commit time to it, and like any new habit or behavior, it may require a little extra effort at first.

Some people go a little too far and have unrealistic expectations about how meditation will affect their lives. They may expect an out-of-body experience with lights and sounds or that their anger will suddenly just disappear. For most of us, these things don't usually happen when we meditate.

Quite frankly, if you look around at a meditation class, what's really happening is that about half the people are actually sleeping. Although you might think this means that meditation is really relaxing, what it usually means is that the people in the class aren't getting enough sleep. So many Americans are chronically sleep-deprived, that is soon as they let themselves actually relax, they fall asleep. If this is a problem for you, you could try doing meditation earlier in the day or use a sitting rather than a lying-down posture. True meditation should be really at the cusp of relaxation when you're still awake and alert.

When you meditate, you want to clear away the information overload that builds up every day and contributes to your stress. The emotional benefits of meditation can include gaining a new perspective on stressful situations, building skills to manage your stress, increasing self-awareness, being able to focus on the present moment, reducing negative emotions, improving your memory and concentration, helping you stick to a physical activity program.

Meditation might also be useful if you have a medical condition, especially one that may be worsened by stress. Some research suggests that meditation can help people manage symptoms of conditions such as anxiety disorders, asthma, cancer, depression, heart disease, high blood pressure, pain, sleep problems.

Science supports many of these findings. For example, researchers at Harvard found that participating in an eight-week mindfulness meditation program appears to make measurable changes in the parts of the brain associated with memory, sense of self, empathy, and stress.

Using MRI images, Harvard researchers actually documented meditation-produced changes over time in the brain's gray matter. For the study, magnetic resonance, or MR, images were taken of the brain structures of 16 study participants. This was done 2 weeks before and after they took part in the 8-week mindfulness-based stress reduction—that's MBSR—program at the University of Massachusetts Center for Mindfulness.

Researchers found increases in the cortical thickness in the hippocampus, which governs learning and memory and in certain areas of the brain that play roles in emotion regulation. There were also *decreases* in brain cell volume in the amygdala, the area that's responsible for fear, anxiety, and stress—and these changes matched how the participants described their stress levels.

In another study at UCLA, researchers found that the brains of long-term meditators were better preserved than the brains of nonmeditators as they aged. Participants who'd been meditating for an average of 20 years had more gray matter volume throughout the brain. Although older meditators still had some volume loss compared to younger meditators, it wasn't as pronounced as in nonmeditators.

In some circumstances, we know that meditation helps, but we're not sure why. A meta-analysis at Johns Hopkins focused on the relationship between mindfulness meditation and its ability to reduce symptoms of depression, anxiety, and pain. Researchers found that among people with depression, meditation produced a response similar to that of antidepressants. This is an interesting finding, and one day, meditation might become part of a care plan for depression. The question is: Why did meditation have the same effect as antidepressants? We don't know yet.

So how does meditation work in the brain and the body? To understand how meditation works, it's helpful to know a little bit about the nervous system.

Practicing meditation has been shown to produce physical changes, such as in the body's fight or flight response. The system responsible for this response is called the autonomic nervous system—sometimes called the involuntary nervous system. It regulates many activities, including your heartbeat, blood pressure, perspiration, breathing rate, body temperature, the production of body fluids, and digestion.

The autonomic nervous system is divided into the sympathetic nervous system and the parasympathetic nervous system. The sympathetic nervous system helps mobilize the body into action—that fight or flight response that we've talked about in previous lectures. The parasympathetic nervous system—or the rest and digest system—slows your heartbeat, allowing your blood vessels to dilate, and improving blood flow. Research is focusing on how meditation may reduce the activity of the sympathetic nervous system and increase that of the parasympathetic system.

Research has also shown that meditation can be an effective way to slow our brain waves—slow down all that traffic in our head—so the body and mind can work in tandem. As each breath begins to lengthen, the brain waves begin to slow.

Dr. Sood, whom I mentioned earlier, says he hears that people think there's only one right way to practice meditation. But Dr. Sood describes meditation like ice cream—there are a lot of flavors, but they all come from the same source, hopefully, a happy cow grazing in Iowa.

As long as you're relaxed in some way, then your meditation practice is a good one. And really, any meditation is good meditation.

With all of this said, you can take the first step toward starting a meditation program simply by setting aside time each day to incorporate some quiet reflection in your life, quieting your mind a little, and focusing on just one thing. That means no multitasking—you can't balance your checkbook and meditate at the same time.

Generally, I find that people these days have a better idea of what meditation is. This wasn't true 10–15 years ago when people immediately thought you were trying to convert them to Buddhism if you mentioned meditation.

About 15 years ago when I founded the Mayo Clinic Integrative Medicine Program, I was convinced of the importance of meditation and tried to get patients to carve out 30 or even 60 minutes of time each day to meditate. It was horribly unsuccessful. People just didn't have that kind of patience; it was too much to ask at once. When Dr. Sood joined the practice, one of the concepts he introduced was to meditate by doing simple things throughout the day.

For example, instead of carving out 30 minutes for meditation, maybe you do 15 minutes of meditation in the morning and then some guided imagery at night before bed. Or you can try some of the simple things he recommends—waking up in the morning and putting your feet on the ground next to the bed and thinking about five people you're grateful for in your life. Or simply silently thinking, "I wish you well," to people you encounter throughout the day. It doesn't have to be one thing and like regular physical activity—you don't have to do all of it all at once.

I really try to impress upon people that it's okay to explore and try different things. I don't want people to feel bad because they weren't able to sit and meditate for an hour. If one kind of meditation doesn't work for you, try something else that may be more your speed—maybe it's tai chi or yoga or going for a quiet walk.

Whatever you can do to try to quiet your mind and let the thoughts flow by, that's what works for you.

For some people, it's really a struggle to keep very quiet, and they get frustrated and think they're not doing it right. Maybe sitting for 15 minutes in silence is a long-range goal, and that's okay. What's important is to start somewhere—no matter where it is—doing something that works for you.

If sitting in silence for 15 minutes doesn't work for you right now, maybe a practice that makes more sense for you is to focus on compassionate thoughts or kind intentions. In these cases, you're not sitting down to meditate; instead, you're being mindful towards the people you meet. That's meditation, too. If you're thinking about starting a meditation practice, here are a few options to start with.

Breath meditation: Breath meditation involves focusing on your breathing, consciously observing every inhalation and exhalation, and the rising and the falling of the chest. Breathing that is deep, slow, and smooth and that comes from your diaphragm is maintained in this practice. The purpose is to slow your breathing, take in more oxygen, and reduce the use of shoulder, neck, and upper chest muscles while breathing—so that you breathe more efficiently.

Mindfulness meditation: Mindfulness meditation is based on the concept of having an increased awareness and acceptance of the present moment. One mindfulness meditation exercise is to bring all your attention to the sensation and flow of air moving in and out of your body. The goal is to focus on what you're experiencing in the present moment without reacting to it or making any judgments about it.

Body scanning: Body scanning means that you focus attention on different parts of your body. Through body scanning, you become aware of your body's various sensations—whether that's pain, tension, warmth, or relaxation. You can combine body scanning with breathing exercises and imagine breathing heat or relaxation into and out of different parts of your body.

Transcendental meditation: Transcendental meditation teaches you to focus on a mantra—a sound, word, or phrase—that you repeat over and over—either out loud or to yourself. The goal is to keep distracting thoughts out of your conscious awareness.

You can create your own mantra whether it's religious or secular. Examples of religious mantras include the Jesus Prayer in the Christian tradition, the holy name of God in Judaism, or the om mantra of Hinduism, Buddhism, and other Eastern religions. For a secular mantra, you can use the words one, love, or peace—or any word or phrase that is meaningful to you. Whatever mantra you choose, it should hold your attention on a single thought or sensation that brings you a sense of comfort.

Analytical meditation: Analytical meditation is when you try to comprehend the deeper meaning of an object you're focusing on. In analytical meditation, you might focus your attention on a scriptural passage or a concept—maybe how precious human life is. Through this type of meditation, the goal is to focus on feeling empathy and compassion towards yourself and towards others. Now that you know about some of the main styles of meditation, here are three types of meditation that incorporate these practices, and how to do them.

Walking meditation: Called *kinhin* in the Zen tradition—with walking meditation, you focus on the subtle movements used to stand and walk. You can use this technique anywhere you're walking, such as in a tranquil forest, on a city sidewalk, or at the mall. When you use this method, slow down your pace so that you can focus on each movement of your legs or feet. Don't focus on a particular destination. Concentrate on your legs and feet, repeating action words in your mind such as lifting, moving, and placing as you lift each foot—move your leg forward and place your foot on the ground.

Guided meditation: Similar to the guided imagery or visualization techniques we discussed in an earlier lecture—with guided meditation, you form mental images of places or situations you find relaxing. Try to use as many senses as possible, such as smells, sights, sounds, and textures. You may be led through this process in a class by a guide or teacher—or you may prefer to use guided imagery programs on your own at home.

Focus your love and gratitude: In this type of meditation, you focus your attention on a sacred object or being, weaving feelings of love, compassion, and gratitude into your thoughts. You can also close your eyes and use your imagination or gaze at representations of the object.

You can make meditation as formal or informal as you like, however, it suits your lifestyle and situation. Some people build meditation into their daily routine—for example, starting and ending each day with time for meditation.

You can also listen to sacred music, spoken words, or any music you find relaxing or inspiring. You may want to write your reflections in a journal or discuss them with a friend or spiritual leader.

When Dr. Sood describes his meditation practice, he says that he starts by thinking of a particular devotion—compassion, health, peacefulness. He says it can become too boring if he just focuses on breathing, so he'll assign meaning to the effort. For example, he might dedicate his meditation to all the babies born today or to children suffering in the world. He tries to think of something that will help the larger community.

Then he thinks of people he wants to invite in, whether it's Jesus or Buddha or Mother Nature. Then he brings his attention back to his breathing. When he gets distracted, he might go back to his devotional focus for that particular meditation, returning his thoughts to the children or the ocean to keep going. He also has a mantra he uses, and he meditates while lying down because that's where he says he can reach the deepest space of relaxation. His whole meditation practice lasts for about 30 minutes.

But even though Dr. Sood's been practicing for decades, he still falls asleep once in a while. So, see? Don't worry about it if it happens to you, too. Don't expect things to go smoothly from the start. Meditation takes practice. Keep in mind, for instance, that it's common for your mind to wander during meditation no matter how long you've been practicing meditation. If you're meditating to calm your mind and your attention wanders, slowly return to the object, sensation, or movement you're focusing on.

Experiment—and you'll likely find out what types of meditation work best for you and what you enjoy doing. Adapt meditation to your needs at the moment. Remember, there's no right way or wrong way to meditate. What matter's that meditation helps you reduce your stress level and feel better overall.

Here are four steps to help you start your own meditation practice: First, find a quiet place with as little distraction as possible. The more often you practice meditation, the easier it will be for you to meditate even with traffic blaring around you.

Next, choose a posture that works for you. Is sitting against a wall comfortable? On a cushion? In a favorite chair? Lying down? They're all fine.

Now it's time to focus your attention. Maybe you want to choose a word to repeat, or you can light a candle and focus on the flame.

The last step is to keep an open mind. Let distractions come and go without engaging them. If they happen, they happen—let them go and bring your attention back to the focus.

My own personal meditation practice varies over time. I often use computer-assisted biofeedback programs when I'm at work—especially if I have just a few minutes here and there throughout the day. I find that seeing my stress level on the screen and watching how I can lower my stress level by focusing my attention and doing some slow breathing—helps me achieve that relaxation response more quickly. I also carry a couple of hand-held biofeedback devices with me when I travel. These are either stand-alone products or devices that can work with my smartphone.

Then, I can turn an unexpected delay at an airport from a frustrating experience to an unexpected opportunity to practice a mind-body approach that's going to help me feel better, lower my stress, and improve my brain. Experiences that used to be frustrating become opportunities. I think the ability to reframe the situations we find ourselves in is a key skill that results from regular meditative practices.

At home, I may meditate one week and then focus on tai chi the next. I'll throw in a few yoga postures here and there as well. The key for me is to keep it interesting and shift my practice based on what's going on in my life. For example, if it's been one of those weeks, and I'm feeling exhausted—I might struggle to stay awake if I try to sit and meditate. So, rather than trying to force myself to stay awake and probably become frustrated in the process—I'll shift to tai chi that day. The gentle flowing motions are relaxing, and I haven't fallen asleep while doing it yet.

At Mayo Clinic, our core value is, "The needs of the patient come first," and we're very aware of the stressors patients face when they're in the hospital. Surgery comes with a lot of uncertainty and often pain as well. Being sick with a serious illness brings similar challenges. As we've already discussed, stress can slow the healing of wounds and reduce the body's immune function—two things we don't want to have happen after surgery or in patients who are trying to recover from serious illnesses.

During the past two decades, we've conducted dozens of studies to try to determine what we can bring to the bedside to help our patients manage their stress more effectively and to feel better and recover faster in the process. We've identified a number of therapies and services that fit this bill. We call this our Healing Enhancement Program.

The Healing Enhancement Program allows us to bring a variety of things to the bedside, so we can try to meet each patient's unique needs. The nurses who provide this service are called integrative therapy specialists, and they're an absolute godsend. They may arrange a visit from a music therapist or one of our Caring Canine teams. If massage is called for, they know who to call to make that happen. But they can do plenty on their own, too, especially when it comes to meditation and other mind-body therapies. These specialists are trained in meditation, guided imagery, and biofeedback-assisted relaxation. I've had a number of patients return to Mayo Clinic years after their surgery and tell me that the mind-body skills that our integrative therapy specialists taught them in the hospital have become an important part of their wellness routine.

We know that our specialists can't get to every room every day, so we also have relaxation options available on our hospitals' Video-On-Demand channels. Patients can tune out the din of the hospital and focus on the waves off the shore of Cape Cod—and either enjoy the natural sounds or listen to music that accompanies the video or even choose to do a guided meditation. We want to make as many options available as possible to meet the needs of as many patients as possible.

I've become a big believer in having patients spend less time watching TV—the evening news isn't conducive to healing, in my opinion, and more time listening to soothing music or sounds or meditating. I've seen a transformation occur for patients and their loved ones when I suggest a switch from war, crime, and politics to a video of the waterfalls of the Fingerlake region of New York. The shoulders drop a bit, breathing slows, and smiles often replace frowns. A similar phenomenon usually happens with the residents and medical students who do rounds with me. They're all working hard in an environment that's very stressful—so when they walk into a room where we have nature sounds playing on a CD or a video of the Red Rocks of Sedona on the TV—the change in their stress level is visible.

This is a good reminder that meditation—and all the good it produces—isn't just for the sick or visibly stressed. It can be helpful for all of us—whether we're recovering from surgery or simply trying to be the healthiest we can be.

In our next lecture, we'll take a look at ways you can put your mind and body to work, as you translate your meditative practice into motion.

Lecture 8

Moving Meditation: Yoga, Tai Chi, and Qi Gong

Meditation refers to a group of techniques that help you focus your attention. For most of the types of meditation addressed in the previous lecture, you're sitting still or lying down. But that doesn't always have to be the case. Moving meditation—another way to focus your mind—follows the same general principles of meditation but adds movement to the mix. Yoga, tai chi, and qi gong are three types of moving meditation. In this lecture, you will learn about how each one works.

Yoga

- Yoga is a series of physical postures—often named after mammals, fish, or reptiles—performed with controlled-breathing exercises. The ultimate goal of yoga is to reach complete peacefulness of mind and body. However, many people coming to yoga today are simply looking to increase their flexibility, relieve stress, or take part in a different form of exercise. You'll get the most out of yoga if you embrace it as part of a whole wellness plan.

- Hatha yoga is a general category that includes most of the styles practiced in Western societies. It includes the practice of "asanas"—the term for yoga postures—and "pranayama," the term for yoga breathing exercises.

- In most cases, hatha yoga is gentle and slow, which makes it great for beginners or for students who are looking for a more relaxed style of yoga that allows them to hold poses longer. Hatha yoga can vary a lot, so it's a good idea to call a yoga studio and ask about what type of hatha yoga is offered before attending a class.

- Yoga and other forms of moving meditation can provide major health benefits. Yoga can lower blood pressure, improve cognition, and decrease anxiety.

- According to Amit Sood, M.D., the head of Mayo Clinic's Mind-Body Initiative, yoga is all about attention. For example, when you're moving your hand, you are completely focusing on that hand and training your attention. You're in the moment and not worrying about life and daily struggles. Ultimately, he says, the purpose of yoga, with its physical postures, is to create a flexible body and a focused mind.

- When looking for a yoga class, you want one that can accommodate your needs. You shouldn't be forced into positions, and you shouldn't feel that you're being pushed past your safe zone.

- Like meditation, yoga also can be used as a short intervention. If you are sitting for a long period of time, taking a few minutes to stand up and do a few stretches can increase your energy level.

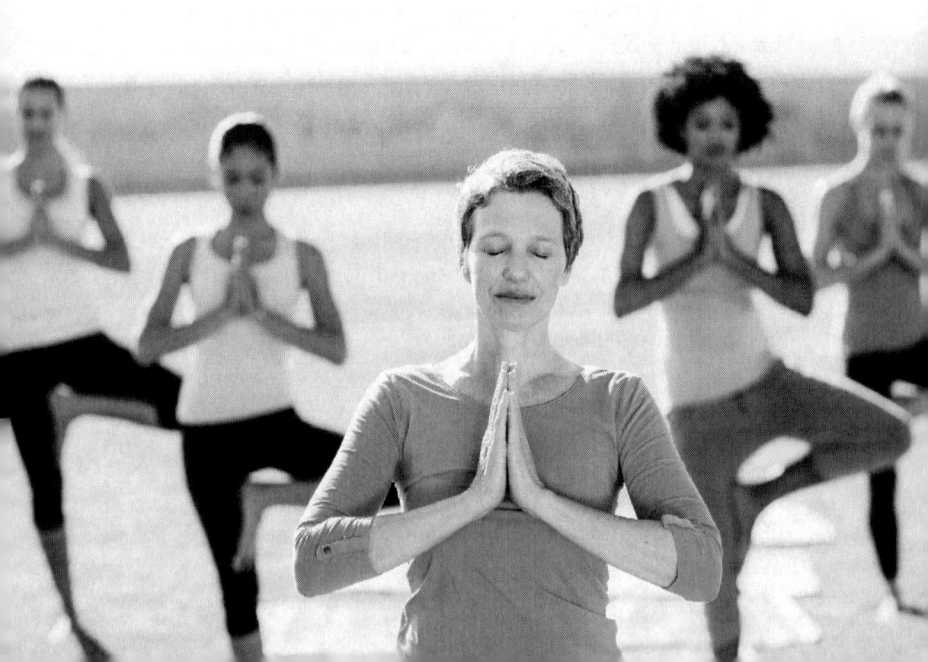

- If you learn a pose or two and practice some stretches or deep breathing, you'll notice some benefit, but you'll get the most out of it if you can invest at least 30 minutes in your yoga session.

- Don't expect too much at the beginning. When you're new, your muscles may be stiff and tight. As you become more comfortable with the practice, you'll reach a point where yoga allows you to recharge your batteries, which helps you feel better and more energized.

- The science says that many people who practice yoga use it to maintain their health and well-being, improve physical fitness, relieve stress, and enhance quality of life. In addition, they may be turning to yoga for specific health conditions, such as back pain, neck pain, arthritis, and anxiety.

- Yoga is helpful in a number of ways, but we don't fully understand the reason behind how it helps. Many studies are trying to tease out yoga's mechanism of action.

- Yoga isn't the answer to all that ails you, however. In studies of certain health conditions—including eating disorders, cognitive disorders, asthma, and arthritis—yoga was used but didn't provide any benefit.

- Yoga is generally considered safe for most healthy people when practiced under the guidance of a trained instructor. But in some situations, yoga might pose a risk. Talk to your doctor before you do yoga if you have any of the following conditions or if any of these situations apply to you.

    - A herniated disk

    - A risk of blood clots

    - Pregnancy

- Severe balance problems
- Severe osteoporosis
- Uncontrolled blood pressure
- Eye conditions, including glaucoma

- You may be able to practice yoga in these situations if you take certain precautions, such as avoiding certain poses or stretches. If you develop symptoms or concerns, see your doctor to make sure that yoga isn't causing you harm.

- Dr. Sood recommends that if you're looking for a yoga class, see if a friend has a suggestion. Make sure that your teacher is credentialed and has some experience teaching people your age and at your experience level. Be careful if a class makes promises about weight loss or if it focuses on herbal remedies.

- The class shouldn't feel competitive, but instead welcoming. The purpose of yoga and meditation isn't about being able to do a handstand or meditate silently for an hour; it's about improving your overall health and becoming a better human being, who is focused and happier.

Tai Chi

- Tai chi was originally developed for self-defense, but it has evolved into a graceful form of exercise. Tai chi involves a series of movements performed in a slow, focused manner and accompanied by deep breathing.

- To understand both tai chi and qi gong, it's important to first understand what "qi" is: a principle of Eastern philosophy that represents the quality or nature of whatever it's applied to. The most specific way to describe qi is to say that it describes the nature, dynamic, and relationships of that which exists.

- The term "tai chi" means "grand ultimate." In Chinese culture, it represents an expansive philosophical and theoretical notion between the balance of light and dark, movement and stillness, waves and particles.

- Traditional tai chi is typically performed as a highly choreographed, lengthy, and complex series of movements. Qi gong, another type of moving meditation, is usually simpler, easier to learn, and more repetitive than tai chi. In tai chi, each posture flows into the next without pause, ensuring that your body is in constant motion.

- Tai chi is a low-impact exercise that doesn't put much stress on your muscles and joints, making it generally safe for all ages and fitness levels. People also find tai chi appealing because it's inexpensive and you don't need any special equipment for it. You can do tai chi anywhere, including indoors or outside, and you can do it alone or in a group class.

- Although tai chi is generally safe, women who are pregnant or people with joint problems, back pain, fractures, severe osteoporosis, or a hernia should talk with their health-care team before trying tai chi. You may need to modify or avoid certain postures, based on what your doctor says.

- When you learn proper tai chi techniques from a qualified instructor and perform tai chi regularly, it can be a great addition to your overall approach to good health. Research shows that tai chi can help you:

  - Manage stress, anxiety, and depression.

  - Improve your mood.

  - Exercise more easily.

  - Get more energy and stamina.

- - Improve your flexibility, balance, and agility.
  - Build stronger and more well-defined muscles.

- Tai chi also may help you:
  - Sleep better.
  - Fight off illness more easily.
  - Lower your blood pressure.
  - Improve joint pain.
  - Improve symptoms of congestive heart failure.
  - Improve your overall well-being.
  - Reduce your risk of falling if you're an older adult.

- You can find many videos and books about tai chi, but to get the full benefits and learn the right way to do it, consider working with a qualified tai chi instructor. Not using the proper techniques can lead to injury.

- To find a class near you, contact local fitness centers, health clubs, and senior centers. Tai chi instructors don't have to be licensed or attend a standard training program, but it's a good idea to ask about an instructor's training and experience and get recommendations if possible.

- After you learn tai chi, you may eventually feel confident enough to do it on your own. But if you enjoy the social aspects of a class, group tai chi classes are out there.

- You may benefit from taking a tai chi class that lasts 12 weeks or less, but if you continue doing tai chi long term and become more skilled at it, you may get even greater benefit.

- You can even practice the soothing mind-body concepts of tai chi without performing the actual movements. Try this when you are in a stressful situation; you may be surprised at the difference it makes.

Qi Gong

- Qi gong, also known as "energy-skill," is an ancient Chinese meditation practice in the tradition of tai chi. It coordinates slow movements with breathing to cultivate your flow of energy, or qi, in a graceful, fluid dance. The movements in qi gong are smooth and rhythmic, teaching balance and increasing flexibility.

- There are two types of qi gong: internal and external. Internal qi gong is a self-directed practice with movements and meditation. With internal qi gong, you control your breathing pattern and work to improve your physical fitness and overall well-being.

- In the traditional practice of external qi gong, a trained practitioner uses his or her ability and knowledge to improve the flow of qi for the person seeking help. A practitioner will use his or her hands to direct energy onto a person's body.

- Qi gong is a form of exercise, but instead of focusing so much on the muscles, it's more of a mindful, energy-based practice.

- Qi gong is focused on stillness, so it can create a very peaceful feeling. In turn, qi gong can help improve concentration and memory. Among its other benefits, qi gong has been found to improve quality of life and reduce the side effects of cancer treatment. It has also been shown to reduce pain and improve sleep, attitude, and mobility in people with chronic fatigue.

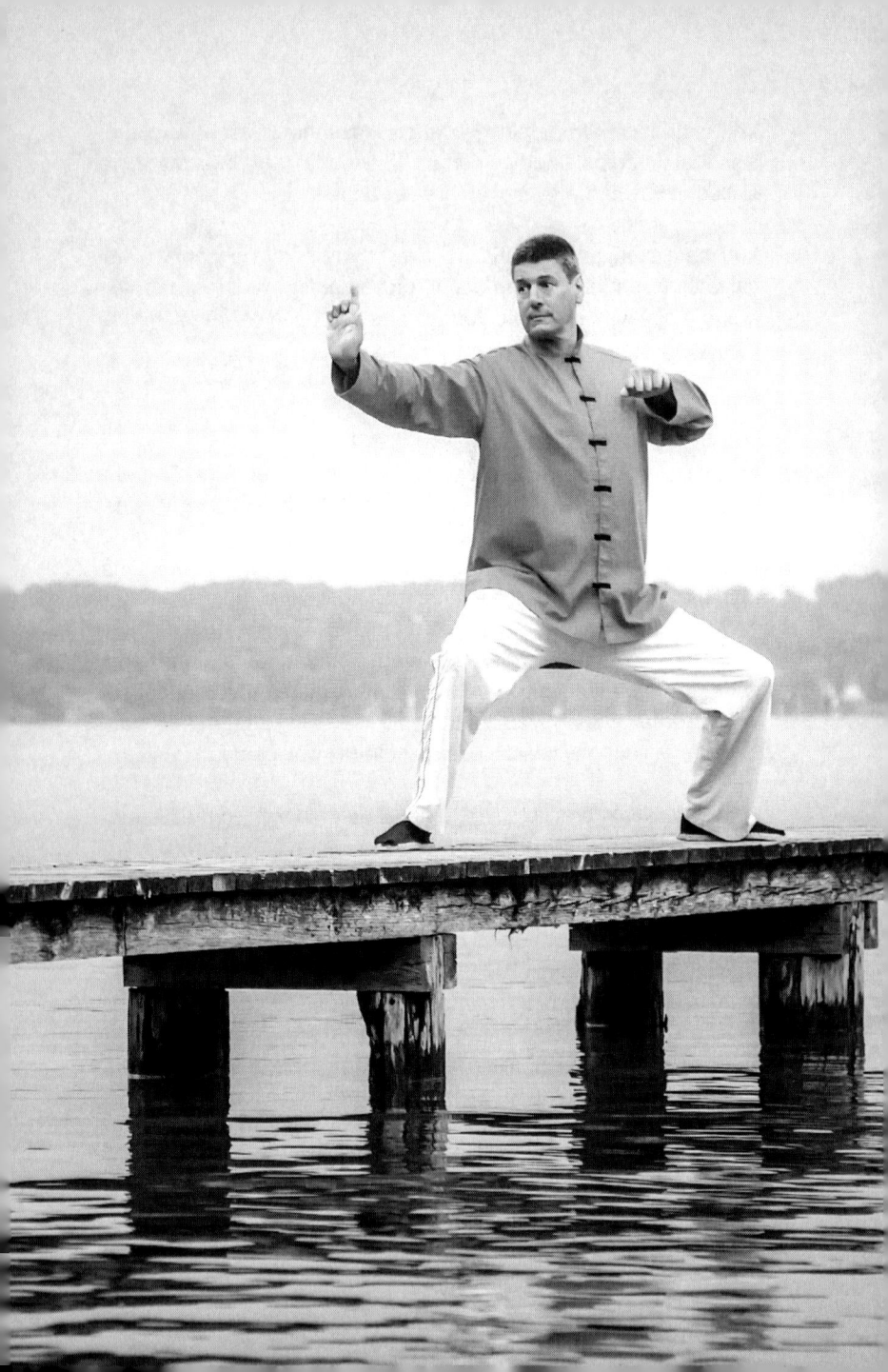

- The strongest and most consistent research on qi gong shows that it can improve bone health, heart and lung functioning, and balance. It also may improve quality of life and self-efficacy (having confidence in your ability to do something important).

- Although there isn't as much research focusing specifically on tai chi and qi gong as there is on yoga and mindfulness meditation, what we've seen so far is promising. A research study conducted by researchers from the University of Minnesota and Mayo Clinic found that external qi gong can help patients' chronic pain.

- Another independent research study found that internal qi gong also relieves chronic pain. In addition to pain, we've found evidence that qi gong may help treat depression—we're just not sure how that works yet.

- How do you get started with tai chi and qi gong? Because both are self-paced and noncompetitive, you don't need a large space to do them or special clothing or equipment. And you can perform them yourself or in a group. Also, because they're both slow and gentle, tai chi and qi gong have virtually no side effects. However, when you're first learning them, make sure that you get proper instruction.

Suggested Reading

Balasubramaniam, et al, "Yoga on Our Minds."

Chan, et al, "A Chinese *Chan*-Based Mind-Body Intervention."

Chan, et al, "Qigong Exercise Alleviates Fatigue, Anxiety, and Depressive Symptoms."

Coleman, "Spring Forest Qigong and Chronic Pain."

Fong, et al, "The Effects of a 6-Month Tai Chi Qigong Training Program."

Gaik, "Qigong as an Alternative and Complementary Treatment for Depression."

"Get the Facts: Yoga for Health," National Center for Complementary and Alternative Medicine.

Jahnke, et al, "A Comprehensive Review of Health Benefits of Qigong and Tai Chi."

Overcash, et al, "The Benefits of Medical Qigong in Patients with Cancer."

Terjestam, et al, "Effects of Scheduled Qigong Exercise on Pupils' Well-Being."

Thomley, et al, "Effects of a Brief, Comprehensive, Yoga-Based Program."

Tsang and Fung, "A Review on Neurobiological and Psychological Mechanisms."

Vincent, et al, "External Qigong for Chronic Pain."

Wang, et al, "Managing Stress and Anxiety through Qigong Exercise in Healthy Adults."

Lecture 8 Transcript

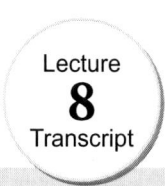

Moving Meditation: Yoga, Tai Chi, and Qi Gong

Last time, we covered many different types of meditation. Now, we're going to keep our discussion of meditation moving—literally. As we learned in our last lecture, meditation refers to a group of techniques that help you focus your attention. For most of the types of meditation addressed in the last lecture, you're sitting still or lying down. But that doesn't always have to be the case. Remember: There's no one right way to meditate.

Moving meditation is another way to focus your mind. It follows the same general principles of meditation, but—as the name suggests—adds movement to the mix. Yoga, tai chi, and qi gong are three types of moving meditation. Let's learn about how each one works.

Yoga hit the U.S. mainstream about a decade ago, but the practice has existed for thousands of years. Now you can find yoga classes at most gyms as well as community centers, schools, and parks. According to the most recent National Health Interview Survey, approximately 13 million U.S. adults and half a million children practice yoga.

Yoga is a series of physical postures—often named after mammals, fish, or reptiles—performed with controlled-breathing exercises. The ultimate goal of yoga is to reach complete peacefulness of mind and body. However, many people coming to yoga today are simply looking to increase their flexibility, relieve stress, or take part in a different form of exercise. It's good to remember that—just as we have seen in the Ornish trial we discussed at the onset of this series—you'll get the most out of yoga if you embrace it as part of a whole wellness plan.

Hatha yoga is a general category that includes most of the styles practiced in Western societies. It includes the practice of asanas—the term for yoga postures—and pranayama—the term for yoga breathing exercises.

In most cases, hatha yoga is pretty gentle and slow, which makes it great for beginners or for students who are looking for a more relaxed style of yoga that allows them to hold poses longer. Hatha yoga can vary a lot, so it's a good idea to call a yoga studio and ask about what type of hatha yoga is offered before attending a class.

Most people start out with hatha yoga because it's fairly simple to learn. But keep in mind that there's a threshold with all new experiences. There are a lot of unknowns, and if you've never done anything like this before or if you're out of shape—it could be intimidating.

What we don't want is for people to assume that they can't do something, or set their expectations so high that they set themselves up for failure. With time and experience, you'll become more flexible, gain endurance, and feel more comfortable.

In return, yoga and other forms of moving meditation can provide major health benefits. Yoga can lower blood pressure, improve cognition, and decrease anxiety. That's a big return for an 8- or 12-week class. We'll talk more about the benefits of yoga later in this lecture.

Dr. Sood, whom I've mentioned in earlier lectures, is the head of Mayo Clinic's Mind Body Initiative. According to Dr. Sood, yoga is all about attention. For example, when you're moving your hand, you are completely focusing on that hand and training your attention. You're in the moment and not worrying about life and daily struggles.

Ultimately, he says, the purpose of yoga—with its physical postures—is to create a flexible body and a focused mind. It's like getting rid of all of our physical energy, so you can focus on your mental needs and not be distracted.

For me, yoga is about joining mind and body. Each specific pose is connected to your breathing and connected to your mind. You're not mindlessly going through the movements. You're focusing your brain on each pose.

A lot of my patients are interested in yoga, but they aren't ready to try a class with a lot of strangers. For patients who feel this way, Mayo Clinic's Patient Education Center has created some basic introductory videos. I give these videos to reluctant patients, so they can go home and try yoga in the privacy of their own home. This taste of yoga is often enough of a door opener—it gives them the chance to experience the potential benefits. From there, they're often ready to engage in more formal training.

In my personal experience, I've found a lot of the yoga poses difficult to do. I struggle with an inflammatory form of arthritis, so my flexibility is limited. Because of this, I don't enjoy a lot of the poses, so I moved to tai chi, which is much easier for me. Again, it's not that there's one right way or a best way when it comes to complementary therapies. It's about finding what works for you and then keeping it as a part of your daily routine. Be willing to try—recognize your own body's limitations—and then find a class and an instructor that are right for you.

When looking for a yoga class, you want one that can accommodate your needs. You shouldn't be forced into positions, and you shouldn't feel that you're being pushed past your safe zone. If you want to go sit on the perimeter while others are doing more advanced poses, you should feel comfortable doing that, and the instructor should allow you to do so. Those are signs of a good teacher.

Like meditation, I think yoga also can be used as a short intervention. When I'm teaching a class or giving a presentation at a conference, we'll perhaps have 250 people in a hall listening to something complex, and I'll see people getting restless. That's when I'll take a three-minute break and have people stand up and do a couple of yoga stretches. I notice that the chatter dies down, and people get reconnected, and the energy level goes up tremendously.

If you learn a pose or two and practice some stretches or deep breathing, you'll definitely notice some benefit. But you get the most bang for your buck, so to speak, if you can invest at least half an hour in your yoga session.

Again, this is about doing what's best for you. Maybe doing 15 minutes of yoga when you wake up and practicing some guided imagery at night will give you the mix that you're looking for.

One more point before we talk about what research says about yoga: Don't expect too much at the beginning. When you're brand new, your muscles may be stiff and tight. As you become more comfortable with the practice, you'll reach a point where yoga allows you to recharge your batteries, which helps you feel better and more energized. Over time, you'll find what's right for you. Maybe 30 minutes of deep breathing, with some poses and stretches and working of your muscles, will give you a feeling of accomplishment.

Many people who practice yoga use it to maintain their health and well-being, improve physical fitness, relieve stress, and enhance quality of life. In addition, they may be turning to yoga for specific health conditions, such as back pain, neck pain, arthritis, and anxiety.

One study funded by the National Center for Complementary and Integrative Health surveyed 90 people with chronic low-back pain. Researchers found that people who practiced yoga had significantly less disability, pain, and depression six months later.

In a 2011 study, also funded by the National Center for Complementary and Integrative Health, 228 participants with chronic low-back pain either took part in yoga, did conventional stretching exercises, or were given a self-care book on managing chronic back pain. The results showed that both yoga and stretching were more effective than a self-care book for improving function and reducing symptoms.

In another 2011 study, this time involving 313 adults with chronic or recurring low-back pain, researchers found that 12 weekly yoga classes seemed to help the participants function better than they did while receiving traditional medical care.

Research also shows that yoga helps with depression. As a matter of fact, there are classes specifically called Yoga for Depression.

Researchers from Duke University analyzed the results of 124 trials on the effects of yoga on people with certain neuropsychiatric disorders, and they found 16 studies that met their criteria. Of those studies included in their review, the researchers found evidence that yoga is helpful in treating depression, schizophrenia, problems with sleep, and attention-deficit hyperactivity disorder in children. In some cases, such as with schizophrenia—yoga was used alongside drug therapy.

The benefits of yoga can even extend into the workplace. Mayo Clinic researchers studied employees who took part in a yoga-based wellness program. Participants met Monday through Saturday for 6 weeks at 5:10 in the morning. Yes, I know that 5:10 in the morning may sound crazy, but bear with me here. At each session, which lasted for at least one hour, class participants did power yoga—a vigorous, freestyle yoga. They also learned about the health benefits of mindfulness, structured breathing, and meditation. As a result of this yoga-based program, participants lost weight, reduced their blood pressure, and reported a better quality of life overall.

So it's clear from research that yoga's helpful in a number of ways, but we don't fully understand the why of how it helps. We've talked quite a bit about the relaxation response in other lectures, and it may be that yoga is simply a good way to activate the relaxation response. A lot of studies are trying to tease out yoga's mechanism of action, but for now, I think we have to live with a little mystery.

Yoga isn't the answer to all that ails you, however, in studies of certain health conditions—yoga was used, but it didn't provide any benefit. For example, researchers studied the effect of yoga on eating disorders and cognitive disorders but didn't find clear evidence of benefit on these disorders. A 2011 review of clinical studies found no sound evidence that yoga improves asthma.

And a 2011 review of medical literature showed that few published studies have been done on yoga and arthritis—and of those that have been done—yoga didn't appear to be very helpful, but it didn't appear to be unhelpful either. Osteoarthritis and rheumatoid arthritis—the two main forms of arthritis—are different conditions, and the effects of yoga may not be the same for each.

The reviewers also pointed out that even if a study found that yoga helped in one way—maybe for osteoarthritic finger joints—it may not help in other ways, such as for osteoarthritic knee joints.

We continue to learn about what where yoga may be beneficial and where it's not. For example, Dr. Mehrsheed Sinaki, who treats patients in Mayo Clinic's Physical Medicine and Rehabilitation department, found that forward bending may cause spinal fractures in people with severe osteoporosis. Once you experience a fracture, your spine may be inclined even more forward, and the risk of a second fracture is even higher. These fractures aren't life-threatening, but they are usually quite painful.

What this means is that if you have severe or untreated osteoporosis, you need to be careful. Check with your doctor before enrolling in a yoga class. And if you do take part in a class, pay extra attention to the postures involved to keep your bones as safe as possible. Forward bends should be done only with a straight back—or stick with lying on your back and keep your legs straight and raising them as far as possible. Your back will stay straight and thanks to gravity and the good carpenter who made the floor, but you'll get all the benefits of a forward bend. My point is, there's always a way to adapt. Don't push yourself.

Which brings me to some cautions. Yoga is generally considered safe for most healthy people when practiced under the guidance of a trained instructor. But in some situations, yoga might pose a risk.

Talk to your doctor before you do yoga if you have any of the following conditions or if any of these situations apply to you: a herniated disk, a risk of blood clots, pregnancy, severe balance problems, severe osteoporosis, uncontrolled blood pressure, eye conditions—including glaucoma. This is a condition you may not think is risky for yoga, but yoga positions—like headstands that put your head lower than your heart—can raise intraocular pressure. That's not something you want if you already have high pressure from glaucoma.

You may be able to practice yoga in these situations if you take certain precautions, such as avoiding certain poses or stretches. If you develop symptoms or concerns, see your doctor to make sure yoga isn't causing you harm.

Dr. Sood recommends that if you're looking for a yoga class, ask around and see if a friend has a suggestion. Make sure your teacher is credentialed and has some experience teaching people your age and at your experience level. Be careful if a class makes promises about weight loss or if it's focused on herbal remedies.

And remember, the class shouldn't feel competitive, but instead welcoming. The purpose of yoga and meditation isn't about being able to do a handstand or meditate silently for an hour. It's about improving your overall health and becoming a better human being who's focused and happier.

Another type of moving meditation that's becoming very popular is tai chi. Tai chi was originally developed for self-defense, but it has evolved into a graceful form of exercise. Tai chi involves a series of movements performed in a slow, focused manner and accompanied by deep breathing.

To understand tai chi and qi gong, which I'll talk about later in this lecture, it's important to first understand what qi is. Qi is a principle of Eastern philosophy. It represents the quality or nature of whatever it's applied to.

In modern times, qi has been thought of as energy because that was the easiest scientific explanation for people in the Western world to understand. That's not quite what qi means—it's not really some sort of energy that you can measure. At its root, the concept of qi comes from Taoist cosmology, a way to explain the nature and order of the universe. The most specific way to describe qi is to say that it describes the nature, dynamic, and relationships of that which exists.

Tai chi literally means grand ultimate. In Chinese culture, it represents an expansive philosophical and theoretical notion between the balance of light and dark, movement and stillness, waves and particles.

Traditional tai chi is typically performed as a highly choreographed, lengthy, and complex series of movements. Qi gong, another type of moving meditation, is usually simpler, easier to learn, and more repetitive than tai chi. In tai chi, each posture flows into the next without pause, ensuring that your body is in constant motion.

Tai chi is a low-impact exercise that doesn't put much stress on your muscles and joints. That makes it generally safe for all ages and fitness levels. It can be a really good activity for older adults who may not otherwise exercise.

People also find tai chi appealing because it's inexpensive, and you don't need any special equipment for it. You can do tai chi anywhere, including indoors or outside. And you can do tai chi alone or in a group class.

Although tai chi is generally safe, women who are pregnant or people with joint problems, back pain, severe osteoporosis, or a hernia should talk with their health-care team before trying tai chi. You may need to modify or avoid certain postures based on what your doctor says.

When you learn proper tai chi technique from a qualified instructor and perform tai chi regularly, it can be a great addition to your overall health approach. Research shows that tai chi can help you manage stress, anxiety, and depression, improve your mood, make it easier for you to exercise, give you more energy and stamina, improve your flexibility, balance, and agility, help you build stronger and more well-defined muscles.

Tai chi also may help you sleep better, fight off illness more easily, lower your blood pressure, improve joint pain, improve symptoms of congestive heart failure, improve your overall well-being, and reduce your risk of falling if you're an older adult

You can find lots of videos and books about tai chi, but to get the full benefit and learn the right way to do it—consider working with a qualified tai chi instructor. Although tai chi is slow and gentle and generally doesn't have negative side effects, not using the proper techniques could lead to injury.

To find a class near you, contact local fitness centers, health clubs, and senior centers. Tai chi instructors don't have to be licensed or attend a standard training program, but it's a good idea to ask about an instructor's training and experience and get recommendations if possible.

A tai chi instructor can teach you specific positions and breathing techniques, as well as how to practice tai chi safely. This is especially important if you have injuries, chronic conditions, or balance or coordination problems.

After you learn tai chi, you may eventually feel confident enough to do it on your own. But if you enjoy the social aspects of a class, group tai chi classes are out there.

You may benefit from taking a tai chi class that lasts 12 weeks or less, but if you continue doing tai chi long-term and become more skilled at it—you may get even greater benefit.

It may help you if you develop a routine and practice tai chi in the same place and at the same time every day. But if this doesn't work with your schedule, don't worry. Doing tai chi wherever you have a few minutes offers benefits, too. You can even practice the soothing mind-body concepts of tai chi without performing the actual movements. Give this a try when you're in a stressful situation, like a traffic jam or a tense work meeting. You may be surprised at the difference it makes.

Qi gong, also known as energy skill, is an ancient Chinese meditation practice in the tradition of tai chi. It coordinates slow movements with breathing to cultivate your flow of energy, or qi, in a sort of graceful, fluid dance. Gong means skill. The movements in qi gong are smooth and rhythmic—teaching balance and increasing flexibility.

There are two types of qi gong—internal and external. Internal qi gong is a self-directed practice with movements and meditation. With internal qi gong, you control your breathing pattern and work to improve your physical fitness and overall well-being.

In the traditional practice of external qi gong, a trained practitioner uses his or her ability and knowledge to improve the flow of qi for the person seeking help. A practitioner will use his or her hands to direct energy onto a person's body.

Qi gong is a form of exercise, but instead of focusing so much on the muscles, it's more of a mindful, energy-based practice.

Qi gong is focused on stillness, so it can create a very peaceful feeling. In turn, qi gong can help improve concentration and memory. Among its other benefits, qi gong has been found to improve quality of life and reduce the side effects of cancer treatment. It's also been shown to reduce pain and improve sleep, attitude, and mobility in people with chronic fatigue.

The strongest and most consistent research on qi gong shows that it can improve bone health, how well the heart and lungs work, and balance.

And there's one more thing about qi gong that I find personally very interesting—it may improve self-efficacy. That may be a bit of an unfamiliar term, but it's an important one. Think of self-efficacy as having confidence in your ability to do something important—let's use exercise as an example. Believing you have the ability to exercise is often the first step in actually exercising. So, I often recommend qi gong or tai chi to my patients who are having a difficult time getting started on some aspect of their wellness plan, such as exercise. Getting a sense of confidence in one area often jumpstarts behavior change in others.

Although there isn't as much research focusing specifically on tai chi and qi gong as there is on yoga and mindfulness meditation, what we've seen so far is promising.

A new research study conducted by researchers from the University of Minnesota and Mayo Clinic found that external qi gong can actually help patients' chronic pain.

Each week for 4 weeks in a row, half of the participants in this study got a 30-minute session of external qi gong treatment from qi gong therapists who were certified international qi gong masters. The other half got a 30-minute session of a different treatment. The study found that the participants who received the external qi gong treatment had less pain.

This study was a randomly, controlled clinical trial. Participants indicated statistically significant reductions in pain intensity in people with chronic pain after their second, third, and fourth qi gong sessions. This finding is especially impressive because most of the participants in this study had been dealing with their pain for more than 5 years.

One of the reasons we looked at qi gong for this study is because managing chronic pain is an ongoing challenge and using medications to deal with the pain isn't enough. Because chronic pain is a part of so many health conditions, we decided to do this study so we could see the effect of external qi gong on chronic pain and so that the results could be generalized on a broader scale.

Another independent research study found that internal qi gong also relieves chronic pain. This study by a nursing school professor at Gustavus Adolphus College in Minnesota found that most of the participants felt much less pain and emotional distress after performing qi gong. Many of the participants in this study also found that they slept better, could concentrate better, were better able to make decisions, had more of an appetite, and were in a better mood when they received qi gong during this study.

The United States government and U.S. military are among the many groups interested in finding better ways to manage chronic pain. In a recent edition of the Gulf War Newsletter, half of the pain management therapies listed in an article on chronic pain were forms of complementary and alternative medicine. Yoga, meditation, Pilates, acupuncture, and massage therapy all made the list.

Likewise, The Joint Commission, a not-for-profit organization that accredits and certifies more than 20,000 health-care organizations and programs in the United States, recently revised its pain management standard. It now specifically highlights the possible benefits of using complementary and alternative medicine such as acupuncture, massage therapy, and relaxation to help manage pain.

In addition to pain, we've found evidence that qi gong may help treat depression. We're just not sure how that works yet.

Psychologist Dr. Frances V. Gaik started looking at low-cost complementary treatments for depression while she was still a doctoral candidate at the Adler School of Psychology in Chicago. She gave 39 patients each a videotape, manual, and audiotapes on qi gong. The participants were asked to do either the exercises or the meditations for at least 40 minutes each day and to keep a log of their practice sessions for 2 months. Dr. Gaik found that participants were able to practice qi gong easily by using these resources.

She also said that as a result of her research, she saw that qi gong was helpful in treating depression—even in people with bipolar depression—and that it helped participants have a better sense of self.

Some of the participants said they were able to cut back on their use of antidepressants, and others found that it helped with anxiety and sleep issues.

Overall, studies have shown that qi gong and tai chi consistently appear to provide positive results for a number of health conditions. For example, in an analysis of 77 studies, researchers wanted to see how meditation exercise affected several facets of health, including bone density, heart and lung function, physical function, fall risk, quality of life, and immune function. The analysis involved more than 6,400 participants across 13 countries.

The researchers found that people who did tai chi or qi gong were able to become more aware of themselves, correct their posture, and pay attention to the movement of their bodies—as well as the flow of their breathing and the stillness of their minds.

After reviewing all of the studies, the researchers identified 163 different health effects linked to tai chi and qi gong. Not all of the studies showed that qi gong and tai chi had a positive effect on health, but a large majority of the studies showed that they did. Here are a few specific examples of what the researchers found.

Qi gong and tai chi had a positive effect on bone health in some cases. This is interesting because most tai chi and qi gong practices don't involve resistance and only some weight-bearing. Traditionally, resistance training and weight-bearing exercises have been recommended to increase bone formation. Qi gong and tai chi were shown to help improve heart and lung function, even when compared to conventional exercise.

So now that you better understand tai chi and qi gong, where do you start? First off, the nice things about tai chi and qi gong are that they're self-paced and non-competitive. You don't need a large space to do them or special clothing or equipment. And you can perform them yourself or in a group.

And because they're both slow and gentle, tai chi and qi gong have virtually no side effects. However, when you're first learning them, make sure you get proper instruction.

In my practice, I encounter a large number of patients who know they should exercise and who want to exercise, but they face hurdles—they're getting older, maybe they're frail, they have some serious health conditions, or they're obese. Many of these patients have heard over and over that they need to get moving, but they can't walk because it hurts their knees or their backs.

For these individuals, a non-impact, gentle approach like tai chi is a foot in the door in terms of physical activity. It's a place for them to start and to gain some sense of mastery, which helps them feel more confident in their ability to overcome barriers on their way to improving their health.

Yoga, tai chi, and qi gong are great examples of how an integrative approach to health can help you. They're three more tools you can add to your health and well-being toolkit. If you want to meet the goals of a N.E.S.S. lifestyle, but are challenged by the exercise portion—being able to perform tai chi, or qi gong may be just the kick-start you need. After a month or two of tai chi, a walk around the block can often become a reality. But even if you don't progress beyond tai chi, by simply doing this type of activity each day, you're still getting more benefit than if you did nothing at all.

I hope this lecture has given you some new insights that can help you find your way forward to a life of greater health and wellness. In our next lecture, we'll delve further into the mind-body connection by exploring relaxation. Until then, best wishes for health and wellness.

Lecture 9

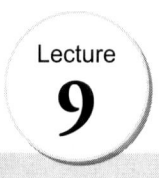

Relaxation Therapies

In this lecture, you will explore several relaxation therapies, both physical and mental, including progressive muscle relaxation, deep breathing, music therapy, and art therapy. With these techniques, as well as the others you have learned about in this course, the goal is to find what works for you as you build the stress management part of your NESS (nutrition, exercise, stress management, and social support) foundation.

Progressive Muscle Relaxation

- Progressive muscle relaxation is a technique that focuses on the slow, steady contraction (shortening or tensing) of a muscle, followed by a gradual relaxation phase, in which you lengthen and release the muscle. The process is then repeated on other groups of muscles in succession.

- When practicing meditation, the idea is to try to get the body as still and quiet as possible. With progressive muscle relaxation, we're also trying to reach a state of deep relaxation, but we do it through tensing and then relaxing various muscle groups in sequence. By doing this, we can identify areas where extra stress or tension is being stored in the muscle and then deliberately relieve that tension.

- Progressive muscle relaxation can help anyone who is experiencing stress. Many patients who are new to the concept of meditation or other relaxation strategies can often start with progressive muscle relaxation and find success with this technique.

- Progressive muscle relaxation is just one more tool in the mind-body tool kit that can help you deal with stress and its effect on your body. The general technique is easy to learn and will become second nature with time and experience. All you need to do is find a quiet spot, some privacy, and some spare moments in the day.

- Beginning with your face, contract the tiny muscles around your eyes, nose, and mouth so that you form a tight grimace. Hold the tension to the count of eight, exhale, and then allow your entire face to become loose and free. You should feel a difference when you do this. You're bringing oxygen to those tight muscles, and then when you let go, the muscles relax.

- You then move down the body, completely tensing your neck, then your jaw, and then your shoulders, holding each set of muscles for eight seconds and then releasing them. You continue this exercise in your chest, abdomen, arms, hands, fingers, buttocks, legs, feet, and toes until all of your muscle groups have been contracted and relaxed.

Getting Started with Relaxation and Breathing Exercises

When it comes to getting started with progressive muscle relaxation and deep breathing, using a CD or podcast or YouTube video and allowing a soothing voice to walk you through each step of the process can be helpful. Some muscle relaxation CDs include a meditative component. Many simply involve suggested progressions of body relaxation, while others incorporate visualization. All of these options can help you achieve muscle relaxation.

The added benefit of using a calming, instructive voice on a CD or video is that a "third party" is there to lead you through each step and help you focus if your mind tends to wander. When you practice these techniques repeatedly, they'll get stored away in your head, ready to access during periods of high stress or tension.

- If you don't have much time, you can do a shortened version of progressive muscle relaxation by applying this technique to just a few targeted areas, such as your face and neck, arms, shoulders and abdomen, chest and buttocks, legs and feet.

- Your larger muscle areas are contracted at once, rather than in smaller groups of muscles. The effect may feel like the gentle unraveling of a tightly sprung coil.

- You can do progressive muscle relaxation exercises anywhere you can add just a few moments of awareness, including in your office or car.

- As with all the other techniques, progressive muscle relaxation won't perform miracles, but research shows that it does have an impact, especially on blood pressure, sleeplessness, tension headaches, and anxiety.

- There haven't been many major studies focused on progressive muscle relaxation, but research that has been done shows that it seems to help people of many ages with many different types of concerns.

- Progressive muscle relaxation is often used with other types of meditation and relaxation therapies, such as guided imagery.

- There are no licensing or certification requirements for teaching progressive muscle relaxation, but many health-care professionals have received training as part of their formal education.

- Many cancer hospitals and clinics offer relaxation training programs that include progressive muscle relaxation. Your health-care team may be able to recommend one for you to try.

- Try to practice relaxation regularly to reap its benefits. If one relaxation technique doesn't work for you, try another. If none of your efforts at stress reduction seem to work, talk to your doctor about other options.

- While progressive muscle relaxation may help lessen your stress, as with other types of complementary treatment, it shouldn't be used as a substitute for standard medical care to treat a health problem. If you're interested in using progressive muscle relaxation to help manage a specific health condition, talk to your doctor about incorporating it into your self-care.

Deep Breathing

- Deep, or relaxed, breathing is a technique that involves deep, even-paced breathing using your diaphragm—the muscle under your rib cage—to expand your lungs. That's why this technique is also sometimes called diaphragmatic breathing or paced breathing. The purpose is to slow your breathing, take in more oxygen, and reduce the use of shoulder, neck, and upper chest muscles while you breathe. This helps you breathe more efficiently.

- With deep breathing, you take a deep breath of air, pause, exhale, and then pause before repeating. This is the most relaxed way to breathe. Your breaths are slow, smooth, and deep.

- Deep breathing can help you relax by reducing the stress chemicals in your brain. It's known to help relieve chronic pain, and some evidence shows that it can help reduce hot flashes that come with menopause, including how often they occur and how severe they are.

- Deep breathing can also help lower blood pressure and decrease anxiety, and it may be useful for chronic obstructive pulmonary disease (COPD). To get the full physical effects of relaxed breathing, it's best to do at least 15 to 20 minutes a day.

- Dizziness, tingling in your extremities, and fainting are all possible on rare occasion with deep breathing. You may want to avoid deep breathing if you experience dizziness or tend to hyperventilate. Otherwise, paced breathing is a generally safe mind-body approach to enhance relaxation.

- Deep breathing releases endorphins throughout the body. Endorphins are feel-good, natural painkillers created by our own bodies. Deep breathing increases the blood flow to your major muscles and makes it easier for your heart to do its work. It's a good way to help your body and mind relax and regain strength and energy.

- The following are some basic instructions to help get you started in trying deep breathing.

    - Lie on your back or sit comfortably with your feet flat on the floor.

    - Relax your shoulders as you breathe.

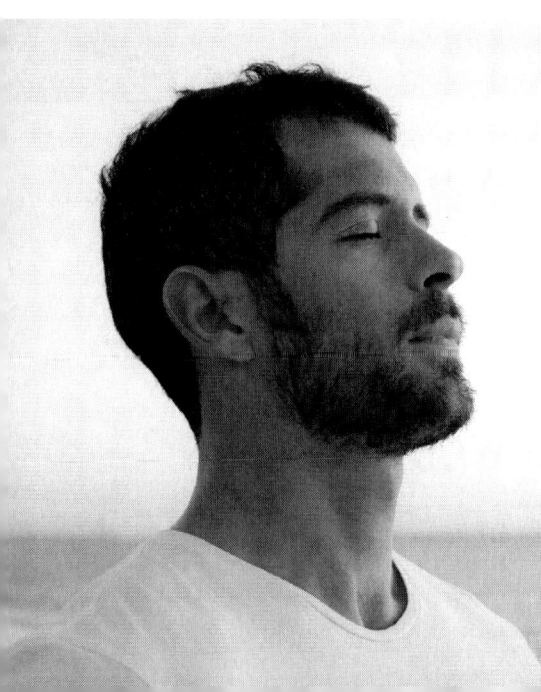

- Breathe in slowly through your nose, allowing your abdomen to expand. Your chest should move only slightly.

- Breathe out slowly through your mouth. Repeat this sequence as many times as you like.

- Focusing on each breath is great for your body in a number of ways. First, if you're truly focused on inhaling and exhaling each breath, you really can't focus on other things. Directing the mind to focus on each breath serves as an anchor and helps prevent wandering thoughts that can be so challenging early in a meditative or other type of relaxation program. Also, the simple act of slowing our breathing produces the relaxation response.

Music Therapy

- Music has tremendous power to help us relax and enjoy life. Listening to music can certainly be therapeutic, but that's not the same as true music therapy. With true music therapy, a trained music therapist works with a patient's health-care team to come up with a plan that uses music therapy to meet the patient's specific needs.

- The therapist is trained to assess a patient's strengths and needs and uses a variety of tools, music, and instruments to help meet the patient's clinical goals. Music therapy can involve creating, singing, moving to, and listening to music.

- Music therapy also provides avenues for communication that can be helpful to those who find it difficult to express themselves in words.

- Music therapists can help people of all ages in a variety of ways. Music therapy has been shown to help lessen the effects of dementia, help reduce the number of asthma attacks in children and adults, relieve pain for people when they're in the hospital, help children with autism communicate better, and help people who have Parkinson's disease improve their motor skills.

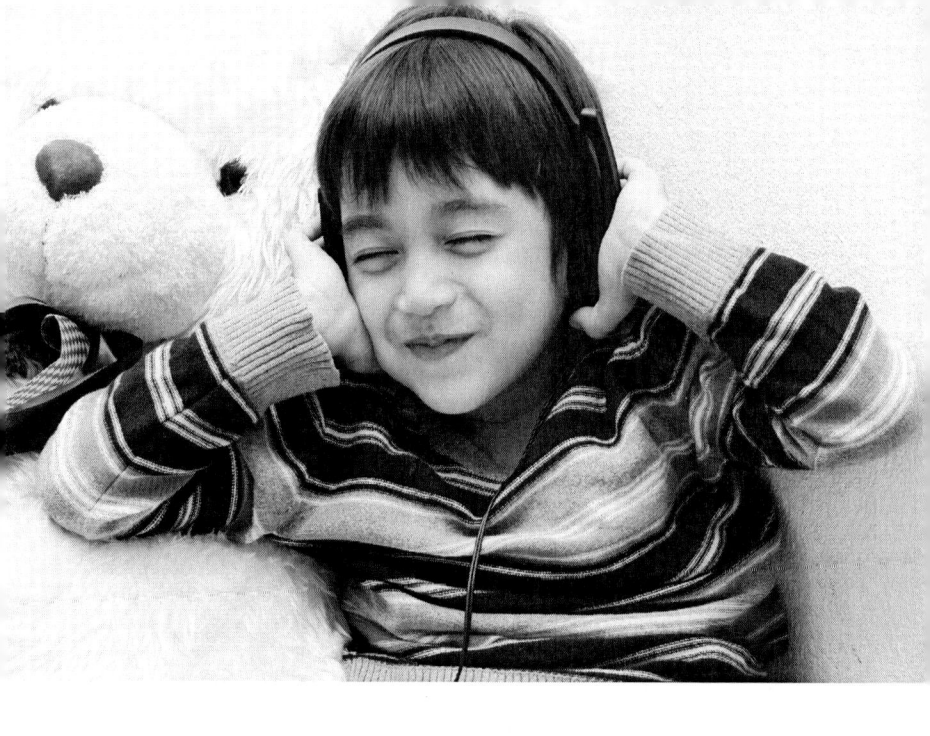

- Music can be therapeutic in more general ways, too. People with Alzheimer's disease who are listening to their favorite songs may feel calmer and less anxious. A piano player in the lobby of a hospital can make everyone feel a little better.

- Finding one specific type of music and using it for every patient population probably wouldn't be successful. In fact, in most music therapy studies or in studies of music in clinical environments, there's almost always an element of personal choice.

- Recorded music is what's used most often for patients who experience music therapy as part of their care; most patients don't experience a live musical performance as part of music therapy. But so far, studies that have been done on music therapy seem to suggest excellent outcomes, even when the music is recorded.

- Music therapy can't replace nursing care, pain medications, or other needed conventional approaches. If you are attuned to music and the appropriate music helps you relax or maybe even fall asleep without the use of medication, then it is worth using.

Art Therapy

- Art therapy is similar to music therapy in that it's based on the belief that the creative process involved in artistic self-expression can help people resolve conflicts and problems and reduce stress.

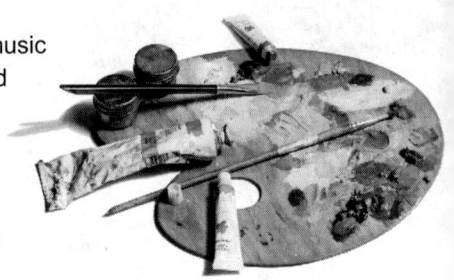

- The uses for art therapy range from helping war veterans to people who have anorexia and people who have experienced abuse or trauma. Art therapy is practiced in a wide variety of settings, including hospitals, psychiatric and rehab facilities, wellness centers, schools, crisis centers, senior communities, private practice, and other clinical and community settings, in both individual and group sessions.

- Numerous case studies have found that art therapy benefits patients with both emotional and physical illnesses. Case studies of young people have involved burn recovery, eating disorders, and sexual abuse. Studies of adults using art therapy have included bereavement, addictions, and bone marrow transplants, among others.

- Art therapy can take many forms, from drawing and painting to pottery and card-making. Getting your hands into finger paint or modeling clay can release pent-up tension and get you in touch with deeper feelings. There are even coloring books and patterns specifically to help with anxiety, where people work with repetitive patterns to help break a panic cycle.

Suggested Reading

Bauer, et al, "Effect of the Combination of Music and Nature Sounds."

Clair, et al, "A Feasibility Study of the Effects of Music and Movement."

Hashim, et al, "The Effects of Progressive Muscle Relaxation and Autogenic Relaxation."

Loewy, et al, "The Effects of Music Therapy."

Mayo Clinic Cancer Center, "A Creative Bedside Manner."

Scheufele, "Effects of Progressive Muscle Relaxation and Classical Music."

Yoo, et al, "Efficacy of Progressive Muscle Relaxation Training and Guided Imagery."

Lecture 9 Transcript

Relaxation Therapies

Today we're going to move into several other relaxation therapies, both physical and mental. Progressive muscle relaxation is a technique that focuses on the slow, steady contraction—shortening or tensing—of a muscle, followed by a gradual relaxation phase in which you lengthen and release the muscle. The process is then repeated on other groups of muscles in succession.

When practicing meditation, the idea is to try to get the body as still and quiet as possible. With progressive muscle relaxation, we're also trying to reach a state of deep relaxation, but we do it through tensing and then relaxing various muscle groups in sequence. By doing this, we can identify areas where extra stress or tension is being stored in the muscle and then deliberately relieve that tension.

Progressive muscle relaxation can help anybody who's experiencing stress. I find that a lot of patients who are new to the concept of meditation or other relaxation strategies can often start with progressive muscle relaxation and find success with this technique. Progressive muscle relaxation is just one more tool in the mind-body toolkit that can help you deal with stress and its effect on your body.

The general technique is easy to learn and will become second nature with time and experience. All you need to do is find a quiet spot, some privacy, and some spare moments in the day. Beginning with your face, contract the tiny muscles around your eyes, nose, and mouth so that you form a tight grimace. Hold the tension to the count of eight, exhale, and then allow your entire face to become loose and free. You should feel a difference when you do this. You're bringing oxygen to those tight muscles and then when you let go, the muscles relax.

You then move down the body, completely tensing your neck, then your jaw, and then your shoulders—holding each set of muscles for eight seconds and then releasing them. You continue this exercise in your chest, abdomen, arms, hands, fingers, buttocks, legs, feet, and toes until all of your muscle groups have been contracted and relaxed.

If you don't have much time, you can do a shortened version of progressive muscle relaxation by applying this technique to just a few targeted areas—such as your face and neck; arms, shoulders, and abdomen; chest and buttocks; legs and feet.

Your larger muscle areas are contracted at once, rather than smaller groups of muscles. The effect may feel like the gentle unraveling of a tightly sprung coil. You can do progressive muscle relaxation exercises anywhere—sitting in your office, in your car, or anywhere you can just add a few moments of awareness. As with all the other techniques we've discussed, progressive muscle relaxation won't perform miracles, but research shows that it does have an impact, especially on blood pressure, sleeplessness, tension headaches, and anxiety.

There haven't been many major studies focused on progressive muscle relaxation, but research that has been done shows that it seems to help people of many ages with many different types of concerns. Here are some examples.

In a small study years ago, 10 women between 60 and 84 years old, who had lost their husbands within the past five years, took part in a 5-month progressive relaxation study. The women, all described as highly anxious, had trouble falling asleep and staying asleep. They also felt anxious and tense and had headaches. After 10 weeks of practicing progressive relaxation, the women all said they felt less anxious, had an easier time falling asleep, and experienced improvement in their headaches.

More recent studies continue to show the benefits of progressive muscle relaxation in a number of different contexts.

Let's take stress as an example. In a 2000 study, researchers exposed 67 men between 18 and 59 years old to a stressful situation and then had them either practice progressive muscle relaxation or listen to classical music or take part in a control group. Participants in the control group either had to listen to a story and write down what they heard or simply sit in silence. Compared to the other participants in the study, the men who did progressive muscle relaxation were the most relaxed and felt the least amount of tension. One way the researchers measured this was by tracking participants' heart rates. They found that the men who did progressive muscle relaxation decreased their heart rates the most. They also had lower levels of cortisol in their systems—cortisol is a hormone that's released in response to stress.

In studies of women with breast cancer, progressive muscle relaxation training has been shown to help reduce nausea, vomiting, anxiety, depression, and even how long women have to stay in the hospital after undergoing a radical mastectomy. Progressive muscle relaxation is often used with other types of meditation and relaxation therapies. In a South Korean study published in 2005, 30 breast cancer patients were trained in progressive muscle relaxation and guided imagery. Thirty other patients in the study received no training. From there, both groups started a 6-cycle chemotherapy regimen.

Researchers found that the patients who were trained in progressive muscle relaxation and guided imagery had less chemotherapy-related nausea and vomiting than the patients who had no training at all. These patients also were much less anxious and depressed than those who didn't receive any training. Six months after treatment ended, the group of women who had received training in progressive muscle relaxation and guided imagery still had a better quality of life than the untrained group.

There are no licensing or certification requirements for teaching progressive muscle relaxation, but many health-care professionals have received training as part of their formal education.

Many cancer hospitals and clinics offer relaxation training programs that include progressive muscle relaxation. Your health-care team may be able to recommend one for you to try.

In general, relaxation techniques involve a refocusing your attention on something calming and increasing awareness of your body. It doesn't matter which relaxation technique you choose. What matters is that you try to practice relaxation regularly to reap its benefits.

Relaxation techniques take practice. As you learn these techniques, you'll become more aware of muscle tension and other physical sensations of stress. Once you know what the stress response feels like, you can make a conscious effort to practice a relaxation technique the moment you start to feel stress symptoms. This can prevent stress from spiraling out of control.

Remember that relaxation techniques are skills. As with any skill, your ability to relax improves with practice. Be patient with yourself. Don't let your effort to practice these techniques turn into one more thing that stresses you out.

If one relaxation technique doesn't work for you, try another. If none of your efforts at stress reduction seem to work, talk to your doctor about other options. In rare cases, the increase in body awareness that comes with relaxation training has led to more anxiety instead of less. Some people, especially people with serious psychological issues or a history of abuse, may feel uncomfortable, emotionally, during some relaxation techniques. If you feel uncomfortable emotionally while doing relaxation techniques, stop what you're doing and consider talking to your doctor or a licensed mental health professional.

While progressive muscle relaxation may help lessen your stress, as with other types of complementary treatment, it shouldn't be used as a substitute for standard medical care to treat a health problem. If you're interested in using progressive muscle relaxation to help manage a specific health condition, talk to your doctor about incorporating it into your self-care.

Deep breathing is similar to some of the meditation practices we talked about previously in this course.

Let's start with some basics. When you breathe, your body takes in oxygen and releases carbon dioxide. When you breathe, you probably breathe mostly through your chest. Your chest rises and falls as you breathe, but this isn't a very efficient way to breathe.

Deep, or relaxed, breathing is a technique that involves deep, even-paced breathing using your diaphragm—that's the muscle under your rib cage—to expand your lungs. That's why this technique is also sometimes called diaphragmatic breathing or paced breathing. The purpose is to slow your breathing, take in more oxygen, and reduce the use of shoulder, neck, and upper chest muscles while you breathe. This helps you breathe more efficiently.

With deep breathing, you take a deep breath of air, pause, exhale, and then pause before repeating. This is the most relaxed way to breathe. Your breaths are slow, smooth, and deep. You're taking only five to seven breaths in each minute. When you're breathing normally, you're taking in 12 to 14 breaths a minute.

Deep breathing can help you relax by reducing the stress chemicals in your brain. It's known to help relieve chronic pain, and some evidence shows that it can help reduce hot flashes that come with menopause—including how often they occur and how severe they are. Deep breathing can also help lower blood pressure, decrease anxiety, and may be useful for chronic obstructive pulmonary disease, or COPD. To get the full physical effects of relaxed breathing, it's best to do at least 15–20 minutes a day.

Dizziness, tingling in your extremities and fainting are all possible on rare occasion with deep breathing. You may want to avoid deep breathing if you experience dizziness or tend to hyperventilate. Otherwise, paced breathing is a generally safe mind-body approach to enhance relaxation.

Deep breathing releases endorphins throughout the body. Endorphins are feel-good, natural painkillers created by our own bodies. Deep breathing increases the blood flow to your major muscles and makes it easier for your heart to do its work. It's a good way to help your body and mind relax and regain strength and energy.

Here are some basic instructions to help get you started in trying deep breathing. First, lie on your back or sit comfortably with your feet flat on the floor. Next, relax your shoulders as you breathe. Then, breathe in slowly through your nose, allowing your abdomen to expand. Your chest should move only slightly. Finally, breathe out slowly through your mouth. Repeat this sequence as many times as you like.

Focusing on each breath is great for your body in a number of ways. First of all, if you're truly focused on inhaling and exhaling each breath, you really can't focus on other things. Directing the mind to focus on each breath serves as an anchor and helps prevent wandering thoughts that can be so challenging early in a meditative or other type of relaxation program. We also know that the simple act of slowing our breathing from 12–14 times a minute, which is what most of us do in a natural rhythm, down to 5 or 6 breaths a minute actually increases our parasympathetic activity and helps balance autonomic function—in other words, it produces the relaxation response.

Now that you know a little more about progressive muscle relaxation and deep breathing, when do people use these techniques? A good example is on an airplane. You're surrounded by people; you really can't spread out. You can't really chant or easily empty your brain in that type of atmosphere. So, if you find yourself tensing up or getting overwhelmed, take two minutes and try some deep breathing or progressive muscle relaxation. The same is true with medical testing. If you're having an MRI and you're anxious about it, structured meditation—like progressive muscle relaxation—is something you can walk yourself through and focus on because it's a little more mechanical.

A minute or two of deep breathing just before giving a talk or presentation can do wonders to help relax and anchor you in the moment. If you're in an argument with your spouse or another family member, even a few deep breaths can help defuse the tension and bring the discussion back to a more rational plane.

Deep breathing can also help you cope with pain or discomfort. In addition to releasing those painkilling endorphins, it relaxes muscles that you've been bracing against the pain—but which really only increase it.

Relaxation breathing can also help with insomnia. I've had a lot of success with younger people who have problems falling asleep—their minds are continually spinning throughout the day. Going through a step-by-step technique helps slow the mind to a more relaxed state.

So how do you get started? Using a CD or podcast or YouTube video and allowing a soothing voice to walk you through each step of the process can be helpful. Some muscle relaxation CDs include a meditative component. Many simply involve suggested progressions of body relaxation, while others incorporate visualization. All of these options can help you achieve muscle relaxation.

The added benefit of using a calming, instructive voice on a CD or video is that a third party is there to lead you through each step and help you focus if your mind tends to wander.

When you practice these techniques repeatedly, they'll get stored away in your head, ready to access during periods of high stress or tension.

And for those of you who are incorrigible multitaskers, you can do both of these techniques—progressive muscle relaxation and breathing exercises—at the same time. As you tighten each muscle group in progressive muscle relaxation, breathe in as you count from one to five, and then relax that muscle group as you breathe out and count down from five to one. Concentrating on doing both techniques well—and in synchrony—should keep you from worrying about your children, your job, and what you're having for dinner at the same time.

Remember that with these techniques, as well as the others we talk about in this course, the goal is to find what works for you as you build the stress management part of your N.E.S.S. foundation. Maybe progressive muscle relaxation will become part of your routine. Or maybe it just doesn't fit for you. That's not a problem—there are lots of other approaches to mind-body therapy you can try.

Most of the techniques we've been talking about so far happen in silence, with a focus on the breath. Our world is full of stimulation, whether it's our phones or the TV or people chattering around us, so many of us find it relaxing just to get away from that constant barrage of noise.

But that doesn't mean we can't find a way to include sound and sight in our mind-body practice. For example, at Mayo Clinic, we incorporate music into medicine in new ways. We've all heard the saying, "Music hath charms to soothe the savage breast," although this is sometimes misquoted as savage beast. Regardless of the original quote, there's no question that music has tremendous power to help us relax and to enjoy life as well.

Listening to music can certainly be therapeutic, but that's not the same as true music therapy. With true music therapy, a trained music therapist works with a patient's health-care team to come up with a plan that uses music therapy to meet the patient's specific needs.

The therapist is trained to assess a patient's strengths and needs and use a variety of tools, music, and instruments to help meet the patient's clinical goals. Music therapy can involve creating, singing, moving to, and listening to music.

Music therapy also provides avenues for communication that can be helpful to those who find it hard to express themselves in words. For example, music therapists worked with United States Congresswoman Gabby Giffords to help her regain her speech after surviving a bullet wound to the head. Music therapists can help people of all ages in a variety of ways. Here are just some of the ways music therapy has been shown to help people. It can help lessen the effects of dementia, help reduce the number of asthma attacks in children and adults, relieve pain for people when they're in the hospital, and help children with autism communicate better.

Parkinson's disease is another area where music therapy has proven useful. In this case, music therapists are working with people who have Parkinson's disease to help them improve their motor skills. Researchers have found that music can help with some of the side effects typical of the disease—shuffling gait, tremors, rigid muscles, and changes in speech. The idea here is that rhythm—like the beat of a drum or the tick of a metronome—can foster slow, coordinated movement when people try to move with the music. Singing exercises and playing kazoos also provide benefit by helping with breath support.

Of course, music can be therapeutic in more general ways, too. People with Alzheimer's listening to their favorite songs may feel calmer and less anxious. A piano player in the lobby of a hospital can make everyone feel a little better.

Music therapy can even help our very youngest people—premature infants. In 2013, researchers at Beth Israel Medical Center's Louis Armstrong Center for Music and Medicine studied 272 premature babies in 11 mid-Atlantic neonatal intensive care units who were 32 weeks or older to see how music affected them.

Researchers examined the effects of three types of music: a lullaby chosen and sung by the baby's parents; an ocean disc, a round instrument, invented by the Remo drum company that mimics the sounds of the womb; and a gato box, a drum-like instrument that mimics the sound of two-tone heartbeat rhythms. Certified music therapists played the two instruments live for the babies. They matched their music to the babies' breathing and heart rhythms.

Although all three types of music therapy helped slow the babies' heart rates, the parents' singing helped the most. Singing increased the amount of time babies stayed quietly alert, and sucking behavior improved most with the gato box—while the ocean disc enhanced sleep. Music also helped lessen the parents' stress.

Clearly, finding one specific type of music and using it for every patient population probably wouldn't be successful. Someone who likes classical music probably wouldn't find heavy metal to be relaxing during a medical procedure and vice-versa. In fact, in most music therapy studies or in studies of music in clinical environments, there's almost always an element of personal choice.

Part of my personal daily stress management strategy is to have classical music playing gently in the background. This doesn't mean I need to schedule a time when I simply focus on the music, but having music in the background often catches my attention. It helps me focus my thoughts while creating a more relaxing atmosphere.

I also often use nature sounds by Chip Davis from Mannheim Steamroller, which he calls ambience therapy. Ambience is the mood or feeling of a certain place. Chip Davis's CDs are nature sound recordings that he makes using special microphones in the woods behind his house.

The music is created with an algorithm that makes a surround sound replay very much like the sounds you might hear in the woods. This can be combined with music, or you can just to listen to the nature sounds alone.

Here's an interesting story: I was listening to one of these nature sounds CDs when I got a phone call from an emergency room nurse. She was in the midst of one of those very busy days that only somebody who has worked in an ER can appreciate.

She started telling me about the most recent case that was coming in for admission, and she suddenly paused. She asked me if she was hearing birds on the phone. I told her I was listening to a CD of nature sounds, and she paused and then asked if she could just listen to the nature sounds for a few minutes, too. She said it was the first chance she had to relax her entire shift and that those 60 seconds made her feel better than she had all day. It was a profound example of the impact that music and nature sounds can have in the midst of a very busy and trying day.

Although we know that music therapy can help people in a variety of ways, we're still trying to figure out how much of a role technology can play in this arena. There's some debate about the role of technology in music therapy. On one hand, if you're listening to a live performance in a hospital room, like maybe someone playing a harp, there's no question that there's something special about the vibrations coming from the instrument itself. Having said that, despite several studies suggesting harp music can be uniquely beneficial for patients, it's not practical to have a harpist and harp in every hospital room.

Recorded music is what's used most often for patients who experience music therapy as part of their care—most patients don't experience a live musical performance as part of musical therapy. But so far, studies that have been done on music therapy seem to suggest excellent outcomes even when the music is recorded.

At Mayo Clinic, we've been using music therapy for our patients in the hospital for many years. Again, the idea isn't that it can replace nursing care, pain medications, or other needed conventional approaches.

If you are attuned to music and bringing appropriate music to the bedside helps you relax or maybe even fall asleep without the use of medication, I consider that a win. Of course, when we have music playing in a room, we see benefits not only for the patient but also for the family members and the medical staff as well.

When I go into a patient's room where the TV is blaring death and destruction and financial crises via the evening news, I can see the negative impact it has on the patient, the family, and even my own team. But when I take that same team into a room where gentle music is playing, or maybe there's a simple nature scene on the TV with soft music in the background, you can really see the difference.

For most of us, music is part of our everyday lives, so it's nice to see that it's finding its way into clinics and hospitals where it can help patients and staff in growing numbers. The German novelist Berthold Auerbach wrote, "Music washes away from the soul the dust of everyday life." That's another quote that reminds me of the value of music therapy.

Art therapy is similar to music therapy in that it's based on the belief that the creative process involved in artistic self-expression can help people resolve conflicts and problems and reduce stress.

The uses for art therapy range from helping war veterans, people who have anorexia, and people who have experienced abuse or trauma. Art therapy is practiced in a wide variety of settings, including hospitals, psychiatric and rehabilitation facilities, wellness centers, schools, crisis centers, senior communities, private practice, and other clinical and community settings, in both individual and group sessions.

Numerous case studies have found that art therapy benefits patients with both emotional and physical illnesses. Case studies of young people have involved burn recovery, eating disorders, and sexual abuse. Studies of adults using art therapy have included bereavement, addictions, and bone marrow transplants, among others.

A 2014 article in the *Journal of Alzheimer's Disease* reviewed research studies on the use of art therapy in Alzheimer's patients and concluded that art therapy engages attention, provides pleasure, and improves neuropsychiatric symptoms, social behavior, and self-esteem.

Many small studies have also been done on the use of art therapy among patients with cancer, Parkinson's disease, HIV and AIDS, diabetes, and stroke with promising results, but more and larger studies are needed. Art therapy can take many forms, from drawing and painting to pottery and card making. Getting your hands into finger paint or modeling clay can release pent-up tension and get you in touch with deeper feelings. There are even coloring books and patterns specifically to help with anxiety, where people work with repetitive patterns to help break a panic cycle.

One example of an art therapy project that can help you deal with stress is called the torn paper collage. It seems to be particularly beneficial if you're feeling like the stresses in your life are out of your control—issues that are interfering with you feeling in charge. The technique allows you to take charge using the art materials. Here's how it works.

Take a variety of colored paper, even old scraps of wrapping paper that you have around the house, scraps of construction paper, pieces of colored newspaper. Begin to tear shapes that appeal to you or use scissors to cut out pieces like tiles, and this will give you more of a mosaic effect. Even when the shapes just fall on the page randomly, they make an interesting pattern. But you can also arrange them very carefully with a certain amount of space in between and get a tiled effect or the effect you would have putting together a puzzle.

When you're ready, and you've decided on part of your image, an area that you like, use white glue or a glue stick and begin to glue your shapes down. Then you can begin to build things around it. You can work abstractly. The beauty is that you're making all the choices here. You're in charge of everything you're doing, which helps reduce stress. It's not about striving for perfection, but rather just enjoying the process of tearing and constructing imagery.

There are a number of small studies done with art therapy that show benefits to patients and staff alike. We conducted a small one here at Mayo Clinic using an artist from the community who came to the bedside of some of our most ill patients struggling with hematologic cancers.

In this particular study, the artist came to the bedside with a number of different media and then asked the patient if they wished to color, draw, paint. But even though many of them claimed to have no artistic talent, almost all of them found some way to express themselves using the various materials provided. And in the process, the experience helped reduce stress and pain and improve their quality of life.

Here are some of the things the patients said: It made me forget all my problems and think about other things totally unrelated to medical problems. It was very enjoyable and lifted my spirits quite a bit. This experience was very lovely. Keeping one's mind on things such as art is very inspiring. Excellent way to remind the patient they are still alive…Yes, you are a person.

Therapies using art and music that tap into our creative energies appear to be beneficial in many ways. They can reduce anxiety, stress, and depression, help with pain management, and even boost immune function in some instances. These therapies give patients an opportunity for self-expression and peace of mind, offering hope and meaning in a difficult time. In our next lectures, we'll explore hands-on therapies, beginning with acupuncture.

Lecture 10

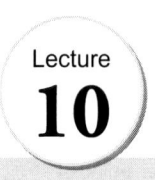

Effective Acupuncture

Acupuncture is a component of traditional Chinese medicine that involves inserting extremely thin metal needles through your skin at certain points on your body. Acupuncture is a technique for balancing the flow of energy, or life force—the qi you learned about in relation to tai chi and qi gong. Those who practice traditional Chinese medicine believe that qi flows through pathways in your body called meridians. By inserting needles into specific points along these meridians, the goal is to rebalance your energy flow. In this lecture, you will learn about acupuncture, as well as acupressure and *tui na*.

Acupuncture

- According to traditional Chinese medicine, the body contains a delicate balance of two opposing and inseparable forces: yin and yang. Yin represents the cold, slow, or passive principle; yang represents the hot, excited, or active principle.

- The goal is to achieve a balance of the two. Disease, in traditional Chinese medicine, comes from an imbalance that leads to a blockage in the flow of qi—that vital energy or life force believed to regulate your spiritual, emotional, mental, and physical health. Acupuncture is meant to remove blockages in the flow of qi and restore and maintain health.

- However, many scientists, physicians, and consumers aren't ready to buy into an energy force that we can't measure or see. So, the more Western approach is to look at acupuncture as a treatment that stimulates nerves and pain pathways, as well as stimulation of the fascia, or the connective tissue fibers.

- Neither theory fully explains how acupuncture works, but it does seem to be an effective treatment, and many studies support its use, particularly when it's combined with other mind-body approaches and Western medicine. But many amazing things have been done with nothing more than acupuncture.

- One of the common misconceptions about acupuncture is that it's a standalone treatment. In reality, acupuncture is usually just one component of a larger treatment program, including recommendations about diet and lifestyle, and it might also include herbs, massage, or exercises, such as tai chi or qi gong.

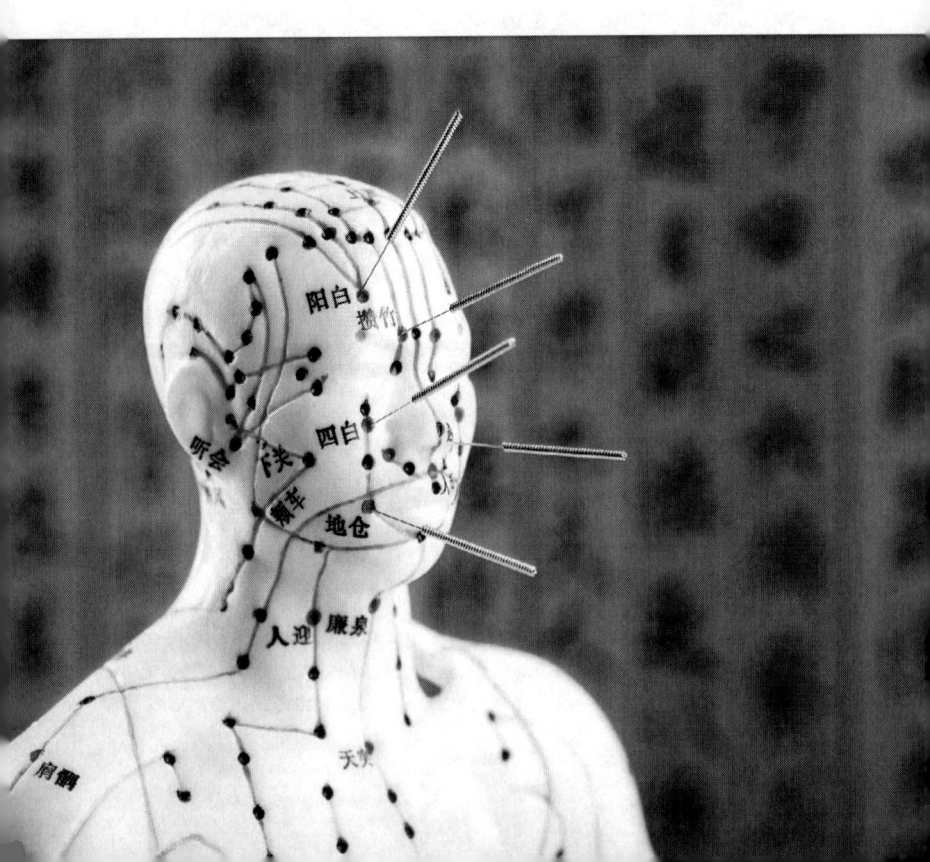

- Many studies have been done just looking at acupuncture in isolation—in other words, taking a group of patients with back pain and providing half with acupuncture and half with sham acupuncture (needles placed in non-acupuncture sites). This is clearly not the way acupuncture would be used in most traditional Chinese medical practices, but even when it's delivered in this suboptimal approach, acupuncture works surprisingly well for headaches, back pain, and nausea.

- While people often link acupuncture to pain control, in the hands of a well-trained practitioner, acupuncture can do even more. It can be effective used alone or when added to other medical treatments.

- The World Health Organization recognizes acupuncture as an effective treatment for a range of medical problems, including:

    o Digestive disorders, such as constipation and hyperacidity.

    o Respiratory disorders, including allergic rhinitis.

    o Neurological and muscular disorders, such as headaches, stroke, and neck pain.

    o Low-back pain and sciatica.

    o Urinary and menstrual problems.

- Most patients experience little or no discomfort with acupuncture. Some people describe a kind of aching or tugging sensation when the needles are manipulated, but this is mild. An acupuncture practitioner will use anywhere from five to 20 needles.

- Unlike therapies such as yoga and meditation, you can't practice acupuncture yourself at home. However, you can get acupressure bands that work for nausea, and you can learn about specific acupressure points. For example, squeezing firmly between your thumb and forefinger may help with headaches.

- Medicare doesn't cover acupuncture, and many insurance programs don't cover it, either. But as the evidence of its effectiveness grows, more insurance companies are taking a closer look at acupuncture. In the meantime, if you're interested in acupuncture but don't have insurance coverage for it, check to see if you have a community acupuncture program in your area. These tend to be less private but often less expensive.

- For most health problems, it may take six to eight treatments to see the full effect of the acupuncture treatment, which is usually given once or twice a week. If you don't see any benefits after six to eight treatments, it probably isn't for you.

- We really don't know how acupuncture works. The classical Chinese explanation is that channels of energy run in regular patterns throughout the body and over its surface. These energy channels, called meridians, are like rivers flowing through the body to irrigate and nourish its tissues. An obstruction in the movement of these energy rivers is like a dam that backs up.

- The meridians can be influenced by the insertion of tiny needles in acupuncture points; the needles unblock the obstructions and reestablish the regular flow of energy. Scientific research to date hasn't found any anatomical structures corresponding to these meridians, nor has anything particular been observed at the classical acupuncture points.

- The modern scientific explanation is that needling the acupuncture points stimulates the nervous system to release chemicals in the muscles, spinal cord, and brain. These chemicals either change how you experience pain or trigger the release of other chemicals and hormones that influence the body's internal regulating system. These responses can occur locally, at or close to the site of application, or at a distance, mediated mainly by sensory neurons to many structures within the central nervous system.

- Our body's natural painkillers—known as endogenous opioids—may play a key role in how acupuncture helps treat pain. Considerable evidence supports the idea that opioid peptides are released during acupuncture, and the pain-relieving effects of acupuncture are at least partially explained by their actions.

- The effects of acupuncture are broad and seem to involve many organ systems, as well as different regions of the brain. The final answer probably will be that acupuncture creates a number of complex, interrelated effects throughout our bodies and central nervous system and that its effects on opioid receptors are just one part of many.

- Treatment for pain is the best-studied aspect of acupuncture. The processing of pain signals involves many parts of the brain, and how much pain you feel partly depends on the context. Research has shown that true acupuncture is better than sham acupuncture in treating chronic neck pain, chronic low-back pain, and acute low-back pain.

- Although we still don't have a complete scientific account of how acupuncture works, we have some pretty good evidence that it does work for certain conditions and for certain people. The number of treatments needed differs from person to person.

- People experience acupuncture needling differently. Most patients feel only minimal pain as the needles are inserted, and some feel no pain. Once the needles are in place, you don't feel any pain. Usually, there aren't any side effects to acupuncture treatment.

- On the day of your acupuncture treatment, there are some things you can do to help prepare yourself. This advice comes from the American Academy of Medical Acupuncture, the professional society of physicians in North America who have incorporated acupuncture into their traditional medical practice.

- Don't eat an unusually large meal right before or after your treatment.

- Don't exercise vigorously, engage in sexual activity, or consume alcoholic beverages within six hours before or after treatment.

- Plan your activities so that after your treatment, you can get some rest—or at least not have to be working at top performance. This is especially important for the first few visits.

- Continue to take any prescription medicines as directed by your doctor. Abusing drugs or alcohol, especially in the week before treatment, will seriously interfere with the effectiveness of acupuncture treatments.

- Keep good mental or written notes of your response to treatment. This is important for your doctor to know so that the follow-up treatments can be designed to best help you.

• If you're considering acupuncture, you'll want to find a qualified practitioner. Take the same steps you would to choose a doctor.

- Ask people you trust for recommendations.

- Check the practitioner's training and credentials. Most states require that acupuncturists who aren't physicians pass an exam conducted by the National Certification Commission for Acupuncture and Oriental Medicine.

- Interview the practitioner. Ask what's involved in the treatment, how likely it is to help your condition, and how much it will cost.

- Find out whether your insurance covers the treatment.

• Although acupuncture has been a life-changing therapy for many patients with chronic pain problems, it can't cure everything. And like all of the other treatments you have been learning about, it still requires that we build our health foundation to see the optimal health benefits.

Acupressure

- Acupressure, sometimes called "shiatsu," is based on the same ideas as acupuncture. But instead of inserting a needle, the practitioner applies physical pressure to specific points on the surface of the body using a finger, hand, elbow, or device. The intent is to restore the flow of life energy, or qi.

- Some people use acupressure simply as a relaxation technique, but it's also used to treat a wide variety of conditions, including musculoskeletal pain and tension, depression, anxiety, sleep difficulties, headache, and nausea.

- Numerous scientific studies support the use of acupressure applied to a specific point on the wrist known as P6 to prevent and treat nausea associated with chemotherapy and surgery, as well as nausea related to the morning sickness that may accompany pregnancy. Some people have found that wrist acupressure also helps reduce motion sickness. The P6 point is located about three finger widths from the large crease in your wrist.

Tui Na

- Another technique that's closely related to acupuncture and acupressure is Chinese massage, also called *tui na*. It's the oldest known system of massage and has been used in China for thousands of years, dating back to the Shang dynasty.

- Unlike other forms of massage therapy, *tui na* uses the meridian system—that's what makes it similar to acupuncture and acupressure. Through the application of massage and manipulation techniques at specific points on the body, *tui na* seeks to reestablish the normal flow of qi.

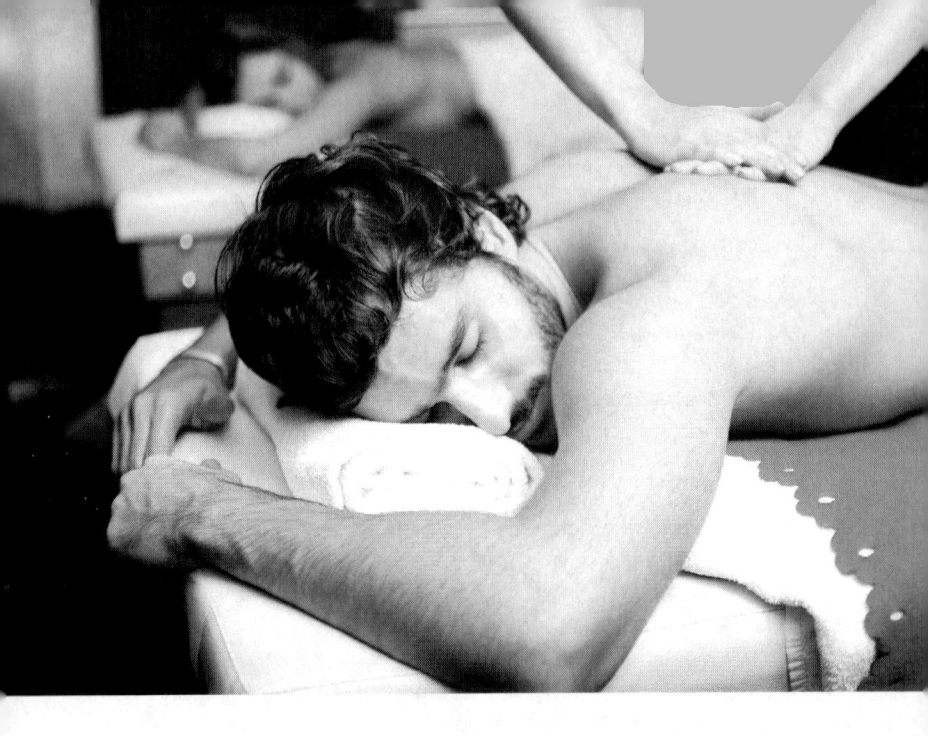

- *Tui na*, which translates into "push and pull" in Chinese, is a series of maneuvers that include pressing, kneading, and grasping, which range from light stroking to deep tissue work. The maneuvers involve hand techniques to massage the body's soft tissues (muscles and tendons). Acupressure techniques affect the flow of qi, and manipulation techniques realign the musculoskeletal system.

- Unlike most forms of massage, Chinese massage generally isn't a light, relaxing massage. It can be very powerful, and some people find parts of the massage to be a bit painful. It's generally used to treat injuries, joint and muscle problems, chronic pain, and some internal disorders. It shouldn't be used for conditions such as a bone fracture or external wound or open sores. It's also not recommended to treat life-threatening conditions, such as a cancerous tumor.

Suggested Reading

Kim, et al, "Acupuncture for Lumbar Spinal Stenosis."

Liu, et al, "Acupuncture for Low Back Pain."

Mallory, et al, "Acupuncture in the Postoperative Setting for Breast Cancer Patients."

Martin, et al, "Improvement in Fibromyalgia Symptoms with Acupuncture."

Suarez-Almazor, et al, "A Randomized Controlled Trial of Acupuncture for Osteoarthritis of the Knee."

Takahashi, "Mechanism of Acupuncture on Neuromodulation in the Gut."

Thicke, et al, "Acupuncture for Treatment of Noncyclic Breast Pain."

"Understanding Acupuncture: Time to Try It?" *NIH News in Health.*

Vincent, et al, "Utilisation of Acupuncture at an Academic Medical Centre."

Zhang, et al, "Efficacy of Acupuncture for Chronic Constipation."

Lecture 10 Transcript

Effective Acupuncture

When I talk to my patients about acupuncture these days, most of them already have some idea of what it is. Like meditation and yoga, acupuncture has entered into our collective knowledge—a big change from just 20 years ago. Acupuncture has become increasingly popular and accepted in mainstream medicine. According to the National Institutes of Health, at least 3 million adults nationwide get acupuncture every year.

Most of my patients already know that acupuncture is a component of traditional Chinese medicine that involves inserting extremely thin metal needles through your skin at certain points on your body. I explain that acupuncture is a technique for balancing the flow of energy, or life force—the qi we talked about earlier in relation to tai chi and qi gong.

Those who practice traditional Chinese medicine believe that qi flows through pathways in your body called meridians. By inserting needles into specific points along these meridians, the goal is to rebalance your energy flow. According to traditional Chinese medicine, the body contains a delicate balance of two opposing and inseparable forces, yin and yang. Yin represents the cold, slow or passive principle. Yang represents the hot, excited or active principle.

Toku Takahashi, a researcher at the Medical College of Wisconsin, suggested this analogy to Western medicine: According to traditional Chinese medicine, acupuncture is believed to restore the balance of yin and yang. This can be translated into the Western medicine terminology that acupuncture modulates the imbalance between the parasympathetic and sympathetic systems.

The goal, in any case, is to achieve a balance of the two. Disease, in traditional Chinese medicine, comes from an imbalance that leads to a blockage in the flow of qi—that vital energy or life force believed to regulate your spiritual, emotional, mental and physical health. Acupuncture is meant to remove blockages in the flow of qi and restore and maintain health.

However, many scientists, physicians, and consumers aren't ready to buy into an energy force that we can't measure or see. So the more Western approach is to look at acupuncture as a treatment that stimulates nerves and pain pathways, as well as stimulation of the fascia, or the connective tissue fibers. At the end of the day, I don't think either theory fully explains how acupuncture works—but it does seem to be an effective treatment, and many studies support its use, particularly when it's combined with other mind-body approaches and Western medicine.

Acupuncture isn't going to fix a severely arthritic knee or mean you don't need to take antibiotics for pneumonia. But a lot of amazing things have been done with nothing more than acupuncture.

One of the common misconceptions about acupuncture is that it's a stand-alone treatment. In reality, acupuncture is usually just one component of a larger treatment program. Most traditional Chinese medicine practitioners take a careful and very detailed history, look at your tongue, check your pulse, and come up with a full plan to restore balance. That plan will likely include acupuncture, but it is also likely to include recommendations about diet and lifestyle, and it might also include herbs, massage, or exercises, such as tai chi or qi gong.

This is an important point when we ask the question, "Does acupuncture work?" A lot of studies have been done just looking at acupuncture in isolation—in other words, taking a group of patients with back pain and providing half with acupuncture and half with sham acupuncture—needles placed in non-acupuncture sites. This is clearly not the way acupuncture would be used in most traditional Chinese medical practices, but even when it's delivered in this suboptimal approach, acupuncture works surprisingly well for headaches, back pain, and nausea.

The concept of sham acupuncture may be a bit unfamiliar, but it's one way of trying to prove that any positive results were in fact due to acupuncture, and not just to a placebo effect. I'll be referring to sham acupuncture more later in this lecture as I talk about different research studies and what they show.

Here at Mayo Clinic, we have a number of dedicated rooms for acupuncture. Our acupuncturists make sure the patient is comfortable. They talk about why they were referred and what they're hoping to accomplish. They make sure there are no reasons why acupuncture shouldn't be used. Then the patient may or may not need to disrobe, depending on which acupuncture points need to be accessed.

We also offer acupuncture throughout the hospital. We might use it to help treat nausea after surgery or to help with the side effects of chemotherapy. While people often link acupuncture to pain control, in the hands of a well-trained practitioner, acupuncture can do even more.

It can be effective used alone, or when added to other medical treatments. The World Health Organization recognizes that acupuncture as an effective treatment for a range of medical problems, including digestive disorders, such as constipation and hyperacidity; respiratory disorders, including allergic rhinitis; neurological and muscular disorders, like headaches, stroke, and neck pain; low-back pain and sciatica; urinary and menstrual problems.

The first question I hear from some patients when I suggest acupuncture is, "Will it hurt?" The answer is generally no. When most of us think of a needle, we're thinking of a hypodermic needle, which is hollow and has a beveled point. That point cuts fibers and tissue, and that's what causes pain. Acupuncture needles are much, much thinner—10 or 12 of them can fit within a regular needle. And they have a beveled tip, so they push the tissue to the side instead of cutting it. Plus, they don't typically go in very deep.

All of this means that most patients experience little or no discomfort. Some people describe a kind of aching or tugging sensation when the needles are manipulated, but this is mild. I've been prescribing acupuncture for more than 15 years and have never had a patient discontinue treatment because of pain from the needles. Of course, I'm also blessed with great acupuncturists at Mayo Clinic who are highly skilled.

An acupuncture practitioner will use anywhere from five to 20 needles. At Mayo Clinic, practitioners also try to create an optimal relaxation response while the needles are being placed. Our treatment rooms have soft music, gentle lighting and, if you prefer, you can watch a video of nature scenes. You'll most likely sit or lie on a special table for 15 or 20 minutes with the needles in place. When you're done, you might feel a little light-headed, but you should be relaxed.

Unlike therapies such as yoga and meditation, you can't practice acupuncture yourself at home. However, you can get acupressure bands that work for nausea, and we can teach people about specific acupressure points. For example, squeezing firmly between your thumb and forefinger may help with headaches.

At Mayo Clinic, employee health insurance covers 12 acupuncture treatments over the course of a year, but that's still relatively unusual. Medicare doesn't cover it, and a lot of insurance programs don't cover it, either. This can be a limiting factor for many people because a single treatment can cost between $50 and $100 or more depending on your location.

But as the evidence of its effectiveness grows, more insurance companies are taking a closer look at acupuncture. In the meantime, if you're interested in acupuncture but don't have insurance coverage for it, check to see if you have a community acupuncture program in your area. These tend to be less private but often less expensive.

For most health problems, our acupuncturists suggest that it may take six to eight treatments to see the full effect of acupuncture the treatment, which is usually given once or twice a week. If you don't see any benefits after six to eight treatments, it probably isn't for you.

So, all that said, how does acupuncture work? As I alluded to earlier, we really don't know how acupuncture works. But let's take a closer look at the current explanations. The classical Chinese explanation is that channels of energy run in regular patterns throughout the body and over its surface. These energy channels, called meridians, are like rivers flowing through the body to irrigate and nourish its tissues. An obstruction in the movement of these energy rivers is like a dam that backs up. The meridians can be influenced by the insertion of tiny needles in acupuncture points; the needles unblock the obstructions and reestablish the regular flow of energy.

Scientific research to date hasn't found any anatomical structures corresponding to these meridians, nor has anything particular been observed at the classical acupuncture points. So what does research tell us about acupuncture? Let's look at some recent studies.

Let's start with a 2010 study from the M.D. Anderson Cancer Center. In this study, researchers tracked 455 patients with painful knee arthritis who received either traditional Chinese acupuncture or a sham treatment. In the real treatment group, needles were inserted at specific points on the body and manipulated in accordance with traditional Chinese acupuncture techniques. In the sham treatment group, needles also were inserted, but not at the locations traditionally used for acupuncture. Compared to a control group, both the real and sham acupuncture groups had statistically significant reductions in pain, averaging about a one-point drop in pain on a scale of 1–7.

So what do we make of this? The modern scientific explanation is that needling the acupuncture points stimulates the nervous system to release chemicals in the muscles, spinal cord, and brain. These chemicals either change how you experience pain, or they trigger the release of other chemicals and hormones that influence the body's own internal regulating system. These responses can occur locally, at or close to the site of application, or at a distance, mediated mainly by sensory neurons to many structures within the central nervous system.

Our body's natural painkillers—known as endogenous opioids—may play a key role in how acupuncture helps treat pain. Considerable evidence supports the idea that opioid peptides are released during acupuncture, and the pain-relieving effects of acupuncture are at least partially explained by their actions.

In other research, Dr. Richard Harris and his colleagues at the University of Michigan have shown that acupuncture increases the number of opioid receptors in the brain. They also found that sham acupuncture didn't produce a similar response. This suggests—in contradiction to the knee arthritis study we just talked about—that while it seemed like acupuncture's effect could occur no matter where the needles were placed, true acupuncture points are uniquely helpful. It's a fascinating area of research, and I suspect we'll see some more definitive evidence, one way or the other, in the near future.

But let's get back to our opioid theory. It seems obvious that if some of the effects of acupuncture are due to the release of our natural opioids, then using an opioid blocker should reduce how well acupuncture relieves pain, right? Well, in studies of patients who were treated with naloxone, a drug that's an opioid antagonist, which essentially means it blocks opioids, the effects of acupuncture were blunted or even eliminated.

Does this mean we have all the answers about how acupuncture works? I don't think so. The effects of acupuncture are broad and seem to involve many organ systems, as well as different regions of the brain. I suspect the final answer will be that acupuncture creates a number of complex, interrelated effects throughout our bodies and central nervous system and that its effects on opioid receptors are just one part of many.

Systematic reviews of studies of acupuncture for low-back pain, spinal stenosis, and neck pain have all been published recently. Researchers looked at 16 studies and found that acupuncture was effective for acute low-back pain in some cases but not in others—but that its effectiveness is stronger for chronic low-back pain. Among people with low-back pain, there was an improvement in day-to-day functioning among people who received acupuncture treatment.

Researchers also evaluated acupuncture specifically in patients with lumbar spinal stenosis and found significant improvement in pain intensity, overall symptoms and quality of life among those who received treatment compared to those who didn't. Spinal stenosis is a particularly painful arthritis of the lower spine where the degenerative changes of the bones and joints actually impinge on the spinal cord or spinal nerves.

However, the researchers couldn't say for certain that acupuncture was effective and safe for lumbar spinal stenosis because the research they studied was limited in scope and may have had a certain level of bias. The researchers also concluded that true acupuncture was better than sham acupuncture in treating chronic neck pain, chronic low-back pain, and acute low-back pain.

Here's another viewpoint on acupuncture: Doctor Richard Nahin of the National Center for Complementary and Integrative Health at the National Institutes of Health says many well-designed studies have found that acupuncture can help with certain conditions, such as back pain, knee pain, headaches, and osteoarthritis.

He says that in many research studies, it's clear that if you're comparing acupuncture to usual care, the acupuncture group almost always does better. The problem is that when researchers compare acupuncture to carefully designed control treatments, the picture becomes more complicated. Well-designed clinical trials need control groups—people who get a sham or simulated treatment called a placebo. Placebos might come in the form of a sugar pill or a saline injection. They give researchers something to compare the real treatment with. But designing a placebo for acupuncture is a challenge.

Dr. Karen J. Sherman, a National Institutes of Health-funded acupuncture researcher at Group Health Research Institute in Seattle, questions whether researchers can come up with a great placebo for needling.

For example, when researchers have compared inserting needles with just pressing a toothpick onto acupuncture points, they've often found both treatments to be successful. But Sherman says many traditional acupuncturists would consider these true treatments as well. The important thing, in their view, is hitting the right spot, not necessarily how deep you go.

Another option for a placebo would be to test a different location. But Sherman says that would be inappropriate for treating pain because acupuncturists traditionally needle tender points. Treatment for pain is the best-studied aspect of acupuncture. The processing of pain signals involves many parts of the brain. And how much pain you feel partly depends on the context.

Here at Mayo Clinic, we've done several studies on how acupuncture affects patients. One particularly successful study looked at acupuncture and fibromyalgia pain. If you or a loved one has fibromyalgia, you know how difficult it can be to manage. One of the most vexing problems is widespread body pain. Unfortunately, it often doesn't respond well to conventional therapies. Since acupuncture has a good track record for treating pain, a group of scientists and physicians at Mayo Clinic hypothesized that acupuncture might help treat fibromyalgia.

To test this idea, they took 50 patients who had been diagnosed with fibromyalgia and divided them into two groups of 25 each. All of them received the usual treatment for fibromyalgia at Mayo Clinic. Then one group received true acupuncture while the second group received sham acupuncture. The research team achieved this by placing a small stand in front of the patient's chest, so the patient couldn't see where the needles were being placed in their arms or legs. The people who received sham acupuncture were given a brief poke by a toothpick without any skin penetration. An acupuncture needle, with its tip embedded into a bandage, was then placed over that point. That way, if a patient happened to look down, he or she would see the needle going through the bandage and apparently also through the skin.

Those who received true acupuncture also had the needle pass through a Band-Aid, but in this case, it actually went into the skin. There is a fair amount of controversy over how best to create a placebo for acupuncture, but at least in this study, when the patients were asked to guess whether they received true or sham acupuncture, about an equal number from each group guessed correctly, suggesting that they were blind to the type of intervention they received.

So basically, they were all treated identically, with the only difference being that one group received eight treatments of true acupuncture. Interestingly, one month later, that group showed a statistically significant reduction in their Fibromyalgia Impact Questionnaire, or FIQ, scores. The FIQ is a standard way of measuring fibromyalgia symptoms.

The patients in this study also had less anxiety and pain. Those results alone are pretty exciting to me since I have many fibromyalgia patients who are in need of better treatments for their symptoms. But here's what makes this study even more interesting: The research team sent the same survey questions to both groups again six months later. The group that received true acupuncture still showed a statistically significant reduction in pain, anxiety, and FIQ scores. Now, this was a small study, so we have to be careful not to overinterpret the results, but there is, at least, some plausibility to the concept that acupuncture could have long-lasting effects.

Researchers at the University of Michigan have found that true acupuncture actually increases opioid receptors in the brain, whereas sham acupuncture did not have that effect. So this, at least, provides a plausible physiological mechanism for why we saw such long-lasting results in the Mayo patients. Although we still don't have a complete scientific account of how acupuncture works, we have some pretty good evidence that it does work for certain conditions and for certain people.

The number of treatments needed differs from person to person. For complex or long-standing conditions, one or two treatments a week for several months may be recommended. For acute problems, usually fewer visits are required. Usually, there aren't any side effects to acupuncture treatment. With the first treatment or two, it's common to have a sensation of deep relaxation or even mild disorientation immediately following the treatment. These feelings pass within a short time and generally don't require anything more than a bit of rest to overcome them.

As I said, people experience acupuncture needling differently. Most patients feel only minimal pain as the needles are inserted; some feel no pain at all. Once the needles are in place, you don't feel any pain. The risk of bruising and skin irritation is less than what you'd experience from a hollow needle. Single-use, disposable needles are now the practice standard—so the risk of infection is minimal.

Patients sometimes ask me if they have to believe in acupuncture—in qi and meridians and so forth—for it to work. The answer is no. Acupuncture is used successfully on cats, dogs, and horses, as well as other animals. These animal patients don't understand or believe in the process that helps them get better. Having said that, a positive attitude toward wellness may reinforce the effects of the treatment received, just as a negative attitude may hinder the effects of acupuncture or any other treatment.

On the day of your acupuncture treatment, there are some things you can do to help prepare yourself. This advice comes from the American Academy of Medical Acupuncture, the professional society of physicians in North America who have incorporated acupuncture into their traditional medical practice. Don't eat an unusually large meal right before or right after your treatment. Don't exercise vigorously, engage in sexual activity, or consume alcoholic beverages within 6 hours before or after treatment. Plan your activities so that after your treatment, you can get some rest—or at least not have to be working at top performance. This is especially important for the first few visits. Continue to take any prescription medicines as directed by your doctor. Abusing drugs or alcohol, especially in the week before treatment, will seriously interfere with the effectiveness of acupuncture treatments. Remember to keep good mental or written notes of your response to treatment. This is important for your doctor to know so that the follow-up treatments can be designed to best help you.

If you're considering acupuncture, you'll want to find a qualified practitioner. Take the same steps you would to choose a doctor: Ask people you trust for recommendations. Check the practitioner's training and credentials. Most states require that acupuncturists who aren't physicians pass an exam conducted by the National Certification Commission for Acupuncture and Oriental Medicine. Interview the practitioner. Ask what's involved in the treatment, how likely it is to help your condition and how much it will cost. Find out whether your insurance covers the treatment.

Don't be afraid to tell your regular doctor you're considering acupuncture. He or she may be able to tell you about the success rate of using acupuncture for your condition or perhaps recommend a practitioner. Each person who performs acupuncture has a unique style, often blending aspects of Eastern and Western medical approaches.

To help determine the type of acupuncture treatment that may help you the most, your practitioner may ask you about your symptoms, behaviors, and lifestyle. An acupuncture practitioner will closely examine the parts of your body that are painful and use several very specific tools to make a diagnosis. The color of your face is one thing the practitioner will pay attention to. Your Western-trained physician is checking this too—a very pale complexion may indicate anemia or shock whereas a very ruddy one might suggest Cushing syndrome; jaundice causes a yellowish tint. But traditional Chinese medicine takes this to a whole new level.

In addition to noting the color of the face, the practitioner may carefully examine the shape, coating and color of your tongue. The tongue is considered an important diagnostic tool in traditional Chinese medicine, correlating certain areas of the tongue with particular areas of the body. Another diagnostic tool, important in both Western and Chinese medicine, is the strength, rhythm, and quality of the pulse in your wrist. Traditional Chinese medicine has an elaborate system of diagnosis based on characteristics of the pulse. An initial acupuncture evaluation may take up to 60 minutes. Subsequent appointments usually take about a half-hour.

Now, moving on to the actual treatment, where will the needles be placed? Acupuncture points are situated in all areas of the body. Sometimes the appropriate points are far removed from the area of your pain. Your acupuncture practitioner will tell you the general site of the planned treatment and if you need to remove any clothing. If appropriate, a gown, towel or sheet will be provided to preserve your modesty. You'll lie on a padded table for the treatment. You may feel a mild aching sensation when a needle reaches the correct depth. Your practitioner may gently move or twirl the needles after placement or apply heat or mild electrical pulses to the needles. There is usually no discomfort when the needles are removed.

After an acupuncture treatment, some people feel relaxed, while others feel energized. But not everyone responds to acupuncture. If your symptoms don't begin to improve within a few weeks, acupuncture may not be right for you.

I have found acupuncture to be an important tool in my treatment toolkit. It's literally been a life-changing therapy for many of my patients with chronic pain problems like recurrent migraines or fibromyalgia. And as the research continues to grow, I find more and more patients with issues that don't involve pain who can benefit from acupuncture as well. But remember, acupuncture can't cure everything—and like all of the other treatments we have been discussing, it still requires that we build our health foundation—N.E.S.S.—to see the optimal health benefits.

Acupressure—sometimes called *shiatsu*—is based on the same ideas as acupuncture. But instead of inserting a needle, the practitioner applies physical pressure to specific points on the surface of the body using a finger, hand, elbow or device. The intent again is to restore the flow of life energy or qi.

Some people use acupressure simply as a relaxation technique, but it's also used to treat a wide variety of conditions, including musculoskeletal pain and tension, depression, anxiety, sleep difficulties, headache, and nausea.

Numerous scientific studies support the use of acupressure applied to a specific point on the wrist known as P6 to prevent and treat nausea associated with chemotherapy and surgery, as well as nausea related to the morning sickness that may accompany pregnancy. Some people have found that wrist acupressure also helps reduce motion sickness. The P6 point is located about three finger-widths from the large crease in your wrist.

Another technique that's closely related to acupuncture and acupressure is Chinese massage, also called *tui na*. It's the oldest known system of massage and has been used in China for thousands of years, dating back to the Shang dynasty. Unlike other forms of massage therapy, *tui na* uses the meridian system—that's what makes it similar to acupuncture and acupressure. Through the application of massage and manipulation technics at specific points on the body, *tui na* seeks to re-establish the normal flow of qi, as we discussed earlier in this lecture.

The term *tui na* translates into "push and pull" in Chinese. It's a series of maneuvers that include pressing, kneading, and grasping, which range from light stroking to deep tissue work. The maneuvers involve hand techniques to massage the body's soft tissues—muscles and tendons. Acupressure techniques affect the flow of qi, and manipulation techniques realign the musculoskeletal system.

Unlike most forms of massage, Chinese massage generally isn't a light, relaxing massage. It can be very powerful, and some people find parts of the massage to be a bit painful. It's generally used to treat injuries, joint and muscle problems, chronic pain and some internal disorders. It shouldn't be used for conditions such as a bone fracture or external wound or open sores. It's also not recommended to treat life-threatening conditions, such as a cancerous tumor.

In our next lecture, we'll take a look at massage therapies and spinal manipulation as they are practiced at Mayo Clinic.

Lecture 11

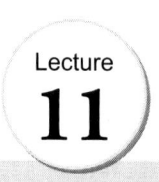

Massage Therapy and Spinal Manipulation

Massage and spinal manipulation are two of the most popular integrative therapies. They are used most often to treat back pain, neck pain, headaches, and arthritis, and they can play an important role in your health and wellness. In this lecture, you will learn about both massage and spinal manipulation, how they work, and where each can help the most. While these therapies are not cures for diseases such as cancer, heart disease, HIV, or diabetes, they may help ease chronic muscle, joint, and back pain and can help you rebound from a sports injury.

Massage

- Massage is a general term for pressing, rubbing, and manipulating your skin, muscles, tendons, and ligaments. Massage therapists typically use their hands and fingers for massage, but they may also use their forearms, elbows, and even feet. Massage may range from light stroking to deep pressure.

- There are many different types of massage. The following are four common types.

    - Swedish massage is the most popular kind of massage. It's a gentle form of massage that uses long strokes, kneading, deep circular movements, vibration, and tapping to help you feel relaxed and energized.

    - Deep massage is a technique that uses slower, more forceful strokes to target the deeper layers of muscle and connective

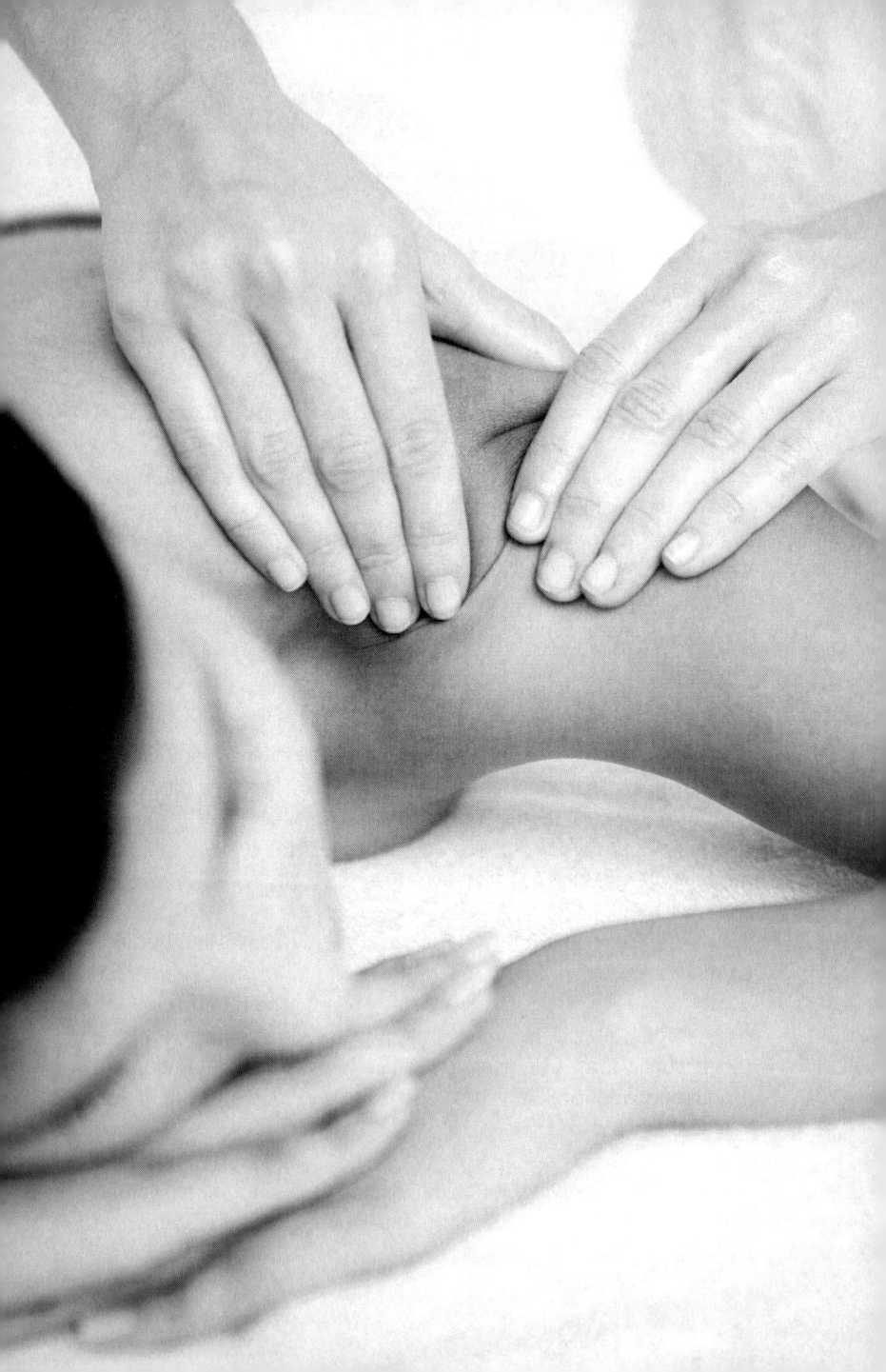

tissue. It's commonly used to help with muscle damage from injuries.

- Sports massage is like Swedish massage, but it's geared toward preventing or treating injuries for people involved in sports activities.

- Trigger point massage focuses on tight muscle fibers that can form if you've injured or overused a muscle.

• Massage is being offered more and more along with standard treatment for a wide range of medical conditions and situations.

• Researchers have found that massage is an effective way to reduce stress, pain, and muscle tension. It releases endorphins—the body's natural painkillers—and increases the blood flow through your body. It can also reduce heart rate and improve how well your immune system works.

• More research on the benefits of massage is needed, but the studies that have been done so far indicate that massage may be helpful for the following conditions.

- Anxiety
- Digestive disorders
- Fibromyalgia
- Headaches
- Insomnia related to stress
- Myofascial pain syndrome
- Paresthesia and nerve pain

- - Soft tissue strains or injuries
  - Sports injuries
  - Temporomandibular joint pain

- Many people wonder why massage has so many profound effects on people. This is a difficult question to answer because there are so many layers involved in massage therapy.

- On one hand, muscles and tissues are being manipulated in a structured and purposeful fashion. Moving muscles and the fibers that connect them might have an impact on muscle pain or alignment or posture.

- But far beyond the simple manipulation of muscle, massage also involves human contact. There's a great deal of power in human touch, and that power is a key benefit in massage therapy. Beyond this, massage usually occurs in a very quiet, pleasant environment; sometimes aromatherapy is also used. The ambience, or the whole effect of the environment, may play a role in the healing power of massage, too.

- No matter which of these components is the main driver—or maybe they all work together—the fact is that most people see very profound effects from massage therapy. They feel less pain, they are less anxious, and their muscles are less tense.

- In most studies of massage therapy, patients say that their overall well-being is improved, too. In addition, a number of studies suggest positive changes to the body, including a decrease in some of the chemicals associated with stress.

- While most people enjoy massage and often feel better after massage—even after a day or two—there's no question that the acute effects of massage generally aren't long-lasting. But even when the memory of your last massage is starting to fade, you may be still enjoying its benefits, even if they're not obvious to you.

- Beyond its specific treatment benefits, massage is something that people enjoy because it often involves caring, comfort, a sense of empowerment, and creating deep connections with a massage therapist.

- Despite this, massage isn't meant as a replacement for regular medical care. Let your doctor know that you're trying massage, and be sure to follow any standard treatment plans you have.

- Most people can benefit from massage, but it's not appropriate for everyone, especially if you have had a recent heart attack, have a bleeding disorder, or are taking blood-thinning medication. If you have deep vein thrombosis, burns, fractures, or severe osteoporosis, massage may be harmful. People with cancer, healing wounds, or nerve damage should avoid pressure on affected areas of the body.

- Be sure to talk about the pros and cons of massage with your doctor, especially if you're pregnant or have cancer or unexplained pain.

- Some forms of massage can leave you feeling a bit sore the next day. But in general, massage shouldn't be painful or uncomfortable. If any part of your massage doesn't feel right or is painful, speak up right away. Most serious problems come from too much pressure during massage.

- No matter what kind of massage you choose, you should feel calm and relaxed during and after your session.

- Several types of health-care professionals—such as physical therapists, occupational therapists, and massage therapists—perform massage. Ask your doctor or someone else you trust for a recommendation. Most states regulate massage therapists through licensing, registration, or certification requirements.

- Don't be afraid to ask a potential massage therapist questions like the following.

    o Are you licensed, certified, or registered?

    o What is your training and experience?

    o How many massage therapy sessions do you think I'll need?

    o What's the cost, and is it covered by health insurance?

Spinal Manipulation

- Another popular hands-on therapy is spinal manipulation, or spinal adjustment. This type of therapy is practiced by chiropractors, doctors of osteopathic medicine, and some physical therapists.

- Research shows that spinal manipulation can effectively treat certain musculoskeletal conditions, such as low-back pain. It's generally considered to be safe, but it's not appropriate for everyone.

- Chiropractic care is based on the idea that your body's structure—nerves, bones, joints, and muscles—and its capacity for healthy function are closely intertwined. By aligning and balancing your body's structure, chiropractic treatment is intended to support the body's natural ability to heal itself.

- Adjustment is one form of therapy that chiropractors use to treat spinal mobility. The goal is to restore spinal movement and, as a result, improve function and decrease back pain.

- During an adjustment, chiropractors use their hands to apply a controlled, sudden force to a joint. This often results in a cracking sound made by separation of the joint surfaces–not, as many people think, by "cracking joints."

- Some chiropractors use instruments to adjust the spine. These methods have not been carefully studied, so their value is uncertain.

- Chiropractors may use muscle pressure and stretching to relax muscles that are shortened or in spasm. Many use additional treatments, such as exercise, ultrasound, and general muscle stimulation.

- Chiropractic care can also be used as a complement or supporting treatment for other medical conditions by relieving the musculoskeletal aspects associated with the condition.

- Chiropractic adjustment rarely causes discomfort and is safe when it's performed by someone who is trained and licensed to deliver chiropractic care. You may have mild soreness or aching following treatment, but this usually resolves within 12 to 48 hours after treatment. Serious complications associated with chiropractic adjustment are rare.

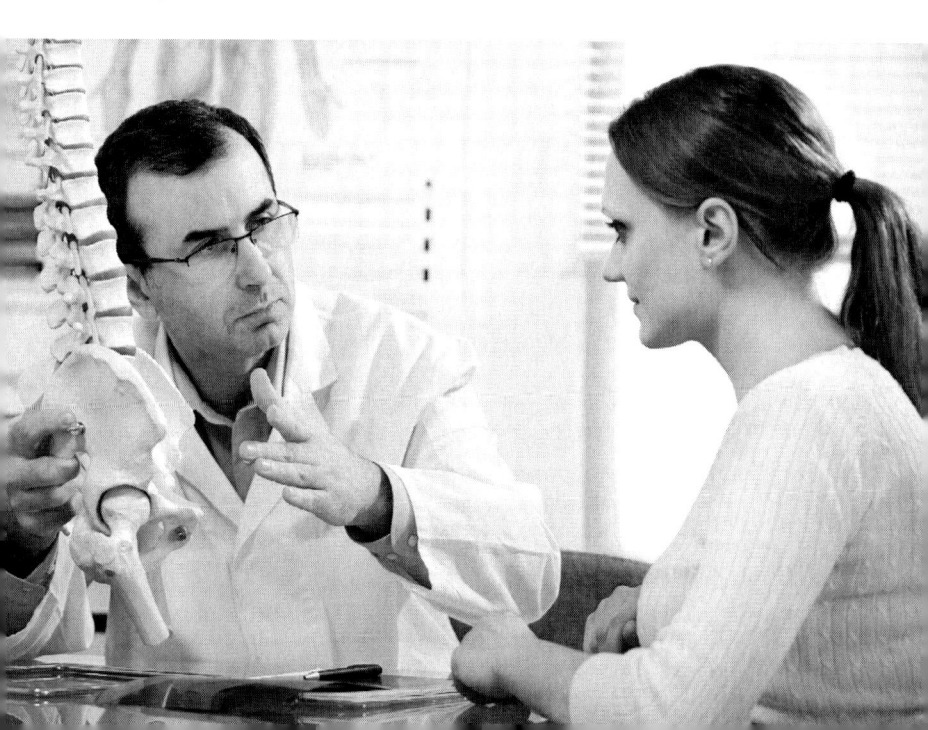

- Don't seek chiropractic adjustment if you have severe osteoporosis, numbness, tingling, or loss of strength in an arm or leg, cancer in your spine, an increased risk of stroke, or an unstable spine.

- Some people experience minor side effects for a few days after chiropractic adjustment. These may include headache, fatigue, or pain in the parts of the body that were treated.

- Not everyone responds to chiropractic adjustments. A lot depends on your particular situation. If your symptoms don't begin to improve after several weeks of treatments, chiropractic adjustment might not be the best option for you.

- Most of the research done on spinal manipulation has focused on back pain, and many studies suggest that it does help.

- In an interview with the *Chicago Tribune*, Ralph Gay, M.D., vice chair of the Midwest Spine Care Practice within Mayo Clinic's department of Physical Medicine and Rehabilitation, addressed the idea of safety within a larger conversation about how medical doctors view the field of chiropractic care. In his interview, Dr. Gay said that medical doctors generally have three main concerns about chiropractic care.

    1. Some medical doctors feel that the education requirements for chiropractors aren't rigorous enough. Unlike traditional medicine, there's no requirement for an internship or residency before a chiropractor is licensed.

    2. Chiropractors don't police themselves very well. State boards regulate practice in all 50 states, but most chiropractors have their own private practice. That means there's not much oversight, and there's not much reason for chiropractors to change the way they practice, even if there are changes they should make.

3. Even if more sessions aren't needed, there's concern that chiropractors keep asking their patients to return. In general, the chiropractic practice model suggests that several treatments over a period of weeks or months is needed to get the most benefit. A trial period is usually six to eight visits.

- But these same concerns could be applied to physical therapy, acupuncture, and massage therapy. Although some chiropractors may look to their business models—more than they do clinical evidence—when they're deciding on a patient's treatment, most chiropractors limit treatment to what's needed for each individual patient based on their response to care.

- Despite these concerns, Dr. Gay said in his interview that he sees medical doctors slowly changing their view of chiropractic care. They're not necessarily referring patients to chiropractors because they have a degree in chiropractic care; they're referring them in circumstances that they feel such care could be helpful and when they personally trust that a specific chiropractor will take good care of the patient.

- In terms of chiropractic care, there are things you can do as a consumer to make sure that you're getting the right kind and amount of care. In his interview, Dr. Gay suggests watching out for chiropractors who recommend initial treatment that lasts more than three to four weeks, who ask for lump-sum payment, or who want to treat you for a condition that's not related to the spine or other common joint or muscle conditions.

- If you're thinking about seeking chiropractic care, be sure to do the following.

    - Ask about the chiropractor's education and licensure.

    - Bring up any medical conditions you have. Ask whether chiropractors have specialized training or experience in the condition you're looking for them to treat.

- Ask how much you'll be expected to pay and if insurance covers your treatment. Chiropractic adjustments are covered by many health maintenance organizations and private health plans, as well as Medicare and state workers' compensation systems.

- Tell the chiropractor about any medications (prescription or over-the-counter drugs) and dietary supplements you take. If a chiropractor suggests a dietary supplement, ask about potential interactions with your medications or other supplements.

Suggested Reading

Bauer, et al, "Effect of Massage Therapy on Pain, Anxiety, and Tension."

Bronfort, et al, "Effectiveness of Manual Therapies."

Clarke, et al, "Trends in the Use of Complementary Health Approaches among Adults."

Cutshall, et al, "Effect of Massage Therapy on Pain, Anxiety, and Tension."

Deardorff, "A Medical Doctor's View of Chiropractic Care."

Dion, et al, "Development of a Hospital-Based Massage Therapy Course."

Dion, et al, "Effect of Massage on Pain Management for Thoracic Surgery Patients."

Dion, et al, "Massage Therapy Alone and in Combination with Meditation."

Drackley, et al, "Effect of Massage Therapy for Postsurgical Mastectomy Recipients."

Dreyer, et al, "Effect of Massage Therapy on Pain, Anxiety, Relaxation, and Tension."

Engen, et al, "Feasibility and Effect of Chair Massage."

Engen, et al, "The Effect of Chair Massage on Muscular Discomfort."

Keller, et al, "Feasibility and Effectiveness of Massage Therapy."

National Center for Complementary and Integrative Health, "Spinal Manipulation's Effects."

Pruthi, et al, "Value of Massage Therapy for Patients in a Breast Clinic."

Rodgers, et al, "A Decade of Building Massage Therapy Services."

Wentworth, et al, "Massage Therapy Reduces Tension, Anxiety, and Pain."

Lecture 11 Transcript

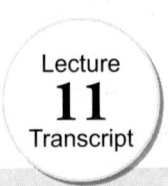

Massage Therapy and Spinal Manipulation

We've have talked about a lot of great therapies and wellness approaches in this course, but now let's focus on one of my favorites, massage therapy. I've not only conducted more than a dozen studies on this particular therapy but also use massage therapy as part of my weekly N.E.S.S. approach.

Massage and spinal manipulation are two of the most popular complementary therapies. They're used most often to treat back pain, neck pain, headaches, and arthritis. At one point in the last century, as modern medicine grew rapidly, hands-on therapies like massage and spinal manipulation weren't seen in as positive a light as they are today. The osteopathic and chiropractic professions in the U.S. struggled for acceptance for years, even as hands-on therapies became part of organized medicine in other countries.

Gradually, these therapeutic tools experienced renewed growth in North America. Today, surveys show that every year, more than 8% of adults use chiropractic care and more than 7% seek massage therapy. Both therapies can play an important role in your health and wellness. Today we'll learn about both of them, how they work and where each can help the most.

Massage is one of the oldest healing arts. It's been used for thousands of years in many cultures to heal, soothe and relieve pain. Massage has been around for a long time through luxury spas and upscale health clubs, but today, it's offered in businesses, clinics, hospitals and even airports. Combined, massage therapy providers represent the largest group of organized complementary care practitioners in the United States and Canada.

If you've never tried massage, today's lecture will give you a good opportunity to learn about its possible health benefits and what to expect during a massage therapy session. Massage is a general term for pressing, rubbing and manipulating your skin, muscles, tendons and ligaments. Massage therapists typically use their hands and fingers for massage, but may also use their forearms, elbows, and even feet. Massage may range from light stroking to deep pressure.

There are many different types of massage. Here are four common types: Swedish massage is the most popular kind of massage. It's a gentle form of massage that uses long strokes, kneading, deep circular movements, vibration and tapping to help you feel relaxed and energized. Deep massage is a technique that uses slower, more-forceful strokes to target the deeper layers of muscle and connective tissue. It's commonly used to help with muscle damage from injuries. Sports massage is like Swedish massage, but it's geared toward preventing or treating injuries for people involved in sports activities. And finally, trigger point massage focuses on tight muscle fibers that can form if you've injured or overused a muscle.

Massage is being offered more and more along with standard treatment for a wide range of medical conditions and situations. Researchers have found that massage is an effective way to reduce stress, pain and muscle tension. It releases endorphins—the body's natural painkillers—and increases the blood flow through your body. It can also reduce heart rate and improve how well your immune system works.

More research on the benefits of massage is needed, but the studies that have been done so far indicate that massage may be helpful for these conditions: anxiety, digestive disorders, fibromyalgia, headaches, insomnia related to stress, myofascial pain syndrome, paresthesias and nerve pain, soft tissue strains or injuries, sports injuries, and temporomandibular joint pain.

At Mayo Clinic, we've been studying massage in a variety of ways. When we first suggested massage therapy for patients undergoing heart surgery, the surgeons were skeptical. All doctors, but especially surgeons, like to have hard data to go on—none of this wishy-washy, feel-good, new-age therapy for them. Prove to us that it works is what they said.

So we did two studies where Mayo Clinic researchers measured the effect of massage therapy on reducing pain, anxiety and tension in people undergoing heart surgery. The studies showed that massage helped reduce pain and decrease anxiety. The proof was in the data. This led the surgeons to hire massage therapists and make massage therapy a routine part of care following open-heart surgery. Then other surgical teams saw these good results, and we soon repeated similar studies in gastrointestinal, breast and thoracic surgery.

The results were so positive that the Mayo Clinic Department of Surgery expanded the number of massage therapists to make massage a routine part of care. Eventually, we expanded massage services to the point that now any of our patients—whether they're having surgery or not—can choose to include massage therapy as part of their hospital care.

Another great massage study at Mayo Clinic was actually led by one of our massage therapists, Liza Dion. Liza had previously worked a great deal with patients undergoing thoracic surgery. So, building on the work that we had done in cardiovascular surgery, we brought massage therapy to these patients. Thoracic surgery is often very painful because the incisions usually involve going through the chest wall. This makes recovery difficult due to the pain that goes along with breathing and moving the chest wall.

The 160 patients we worked with during their recovery from thoracic surgery all received individualized massage therapy. By this, I mean that the massage therapist was able to interview each patient, outline goals, find out where the patient had the most symptoms and then apply massage in the way that the massage therapist felt best suited the circumstances.

I like this type of study because I think it's more true to the actual process of massage therapy in the real world. Some other research trials have tried to make the process very uniform so that there's less variability in the experiment. Sometimes they'll ask the massage therapist only to work on certain areas of the body or spend required amounts of time on each arm or each leg. This gets rid of some variability in the research, but in the process, it destroys some of the true power of massage therapy. What we found in this particular study was that patients reported dramatically lower levels of pain—a statistically significant change.

Here's another interesting note: For this research, we were careful to talk to our staff nurses and physicians to find out if having massage therapists working with patients on the floor might interfere with patient care. We learned that, in fact, it was just the opposite. Many nurses commented that patients who had been anxious or were having difficulty felt so much better with massage—in essence, massage made these patients easier to care for.

As with other studies we've done at Mayo Clinic, we asked patients for their comments because sometimes what we hear directly from patients is more powerful than the P value in standard deviations. One patient said, "Massage is what's getting me through my medical crisis." Another patient said, "I feel I can breathe again." These patients weren't ready to give up their narcotic treatment or other conventional approaches to pain management, but it's clear that all of them gained something from massage. I think it's great that we can bring a simple, noninvasive, safe practice like massage to the bedside. This is another example of integrating the best of both worlds by using evidence in a thoughtful approach.

Not all of our studies in massage focused on surgical patients. Another study, led by one of our cardiac nurses, looked at the effects of a 20-minute massage on patients getting ready to have an invasive cardiovascular procedure. We had 130 patients who were getting ready for cardiac catheterization and divided them into two groups. One group received 20 minutes of hands-on massage at least 30 minutes before the procedure; the other group of patients just received routine care. We used standard rating tools to measure patients' pain, anxiety and muscle tension. The group that received massage showed statistically significant improvement in their levels of pain, anxiety, tension, and even overall satisfaction.

If you've ever been through a cardiac catheterization, you know how stressful it can be. If you haven't, just imagine lying on a large table with a lot of high-tech machinery, and all around you a group of people, working quickly and efficiently, are preparing to place a small catheter into your groin and thread it up through the vessels into your heart. Just thinking about it makes most people a bit nervous. Keep in mind everything we've been saying about stress. If you're getting ready to undergo a procedure like this, it's not in your best interest to be experiencing a lot of stress at that time. That's why bringing massage to patients before they undergo a procedure like this makes sense.

Not all of our studies focus solely on patients. As we did more and more studies on the hospital floors, more and more of our staff came to us and asked, "When is it our turn?" What they were bringing to our attention is that it's very stressful to work in a hospital environment these days. Patients tend to be sicker than ever. They often have many different problems at the same time, and the increased demands for documentation make working in a hospital very stressful.

That led us to do a pilot trial, using chair massage for nurses working in the highly stressful environments of our fibromyalgia unit or in the inpatient psychiatric unit. For this trial, nurses were given a 15-minute chair massage. We saw a dramatic decrease in stress-related symptoms and anxiety, and almost 80% of the nurses said they felt that their overall job satisfaction improved because of massages. Again, this simple study seems to point us in an easy direction.

Many people ask me why massage has so many profound effects on people. I think this is a hard question to answer because there are so many layers involved in massage therapy. On the one hand, muscles and tissues are being manipulated in a structured and purposeful fashion. Moving muscles and the fibers that connect them might have an impact on muscle pain or alignment or posture.

But far beyond the simple manipulation of muscle, massage also involves human contact. There's a great deal of power in human touch. Think about being sick as a child and your mother laying her hand across your fevered brow. Even a gentle kiss from Mom often took the sting out of a scrape or cut. That power of touch is definitely a key benefit in massage therapy.

Beyond this, massage usually occurs in a very quiet, pleasant environment; sometimes aromatherapy is also used. You'll often hear pleasant and relaxing music, and the room may have natural treatments or plants or other things that may induce thoughts of health and healing. The point here is that the ambience or the whole effect of the environment may play a role in the healing power of massage, too.

No matter which of these components is the main driver—or maybe they all work together—the fact is that most people see very profound effects from massage therapy. They feel less pain, they're less anxious, and their muscles are less tense. In most studies of massage therapy, patients say their overall well-being is improved, too. We also have a number of studies that suggest positive changes to the body, including a decrease in some of the chemicals associated with stress, like cortisol.

While most people enjoy massage and often feel better after massage—even after a day or two—there's no question that the acute effects of massage generally aren't long-lasting. But even when the memory of your last massage is starting to fade, you may be still enjoying its benefits, even if they're not obvious to you.

Beyond its specific treatment benefits, massage is something that people enjoy because it often involves caring, comfort, a sense of empowerment, and creating deep connections with a massage therapist. Despite this, massage isn't meant as a replacement for regular medical care. Let your doctor know you're trying massage and be sure to follow any standard treatment plans you have.

Most people can benefit from massage—but it's not appropriate for everyone, especially if you have had a recent heart attack, have a bleeding disorder, or are taking blood-thinning medication. If you have deep vein thrombosis, burns, fractures, or severe osteoporosis, massage may be harmful. People with cancer, healing wounds or nerve damage should avoid pressure on affected areas of the body. Be sure to talk about the pros and cons of massage with your doctor, especially if you're pregnant or have cancer or unexplained pain.

Some forms of massage can leave you feeling a bit sore the next day. But in general, massage shouldn't be painful or uncomfortable. If any part of your massage doesn't feel right or is painful, speak up right away. Most serious problems come from too much pressure during massage.

No matter what kind of massage you choose, you should feel calm and relaxed during and after your session. When you have a massage, here's what to expect: You'll likely need to answer a few questions. Your massage therapist will want to know what you hope to gain from your massage. For example, are you looking for help with a pulled muscle? Your massage therapist will also want to know about any medical conditions you might have.

You may need to undress or wear loose-fitting clothing. Undress only to the point that you're comfortable. You generally lie on a table and cover yourself with a sheet. Most of the time, you start by lying on your stomach and then flip over halfway through. The therapist may use pillows or bolsters to take strain off your lower back and allow you to relax completely during the massage. You can also have a massage while sitting in a chair that's specially made to slope forward so the therapist can work on your back while you're fully clothed. Your massage therapist should perform an evaluation through touch to locate painful or tense areas and to determine how much pressure to apply.

Depending on preference, your massage therapist may use oil or lotion to reduce friction on your skin. Tell your massage therapist if you might be allergic to any ingredients or are sensitive to certain scents. Your massage session may last from 15–90 minutes, depending on the type of massage and how much time you have. No matter what kind of massage you choose, you should feel calm and relaxed during and after your massage.

Finally, as I mentioned earlier, you shouldn't feel significant pain during a massage. If a massage therapist is pushing too hard, ask for lighter pressure. Occasionally you may have a sensitive spot in a muscle that feels like a knot. It's likely to be uncomfortable while your massage therapist works it out. But if it becomes painful, speak up.

Several types of health care professionals—such as physical therapists, occupational therapists, and massage therapists—perform massage. Ask your doctor or someone else you trust for a recommendation. Most states regulate massage therapists through licensing, registration or certification requirements. Don't be afraid to ask a potential massage therapist questions like these: Are you licensed, certified or registered? What is your training and experience? How many massage therapy sessions do you think I'll need? What's the cost, and is it covered by health insurance?

Another popular hands-on therapy is spinal manipulation or spinal adjustment. This type of therapy is practiced by chiropractors, doctors of osteopathic medicine and some physical therapists. Research shows that spinal manipulation can effectively treat certain musculoskeletal conditions, such as low-back pain. It's generally considered to be safe, but it's not appropriate for everyone.

Chiropractic care is based on the idea that your body's structure—nerves, bones, joints and muscles—and its capacity for healthy function are closely intertwined. By aligning and balancing your body's structure, chiropractic treatment is intended to support the body's natural ability to heal itself.

The term "chiropractic" combines the Greek words *cheir*, meaning hand and *praxis*, which means practice to describe a treatment done by hand. According to the 2012 National Health Interview Survey, about 8.4% of adults—more than 19 million—had received chiropractic care in the past 12 months. This survey also shows that Americans spent $4 billion out of their own pockets on visits to practitioners of chiropractic or osteopathic manipulation. Adjustment is one form of therapy chiropractors use to treat spinal mobility. The goal is to restore spinal movement and, as a result, improve function and decrease back pain. During an adjustment, chiropractors use their hands to apply a controlled, sudden force to a joint. This often results in a cracking sound made by separation of the joint surfaces—not, as many people think, by cracking joints.

Some chiropractors use instruments to adjust the spine. These methods have not been carefully studied, so their value is uncertain. Chiropractors may use muscle pressure and stretching to relax muscles that are shortened or in spasm. Many use additional treatments such as exercise, ultrasound, and general muscle stimulation.

According to the American Chiropractic Association, people often go to chiropractors for neuromusculoskeletal issues, such as headaches, joint pain, neck pain, low-back pain, and sciatica. Chiropractors also treat patients with osteoarthritis, spinal disk conditions, carpal tunnel syndrome, tendonitis, sprains, and strains.

Tissue injury may be caused by a single traumatic event, such as improper lifting of a heavy object, or through repetitive stresses, such as sitting in an awkward position with poor spinal posture for an extended period of time. In either case, injury leads to physical and chemical changes that can cause inflammation, pain, and loss of function. Manipulating or adjusting the affected joints and tissues can help you move those joints more easily and can help relieve pain and muscle tightness while your tissues heal.

Chiropractic care can also be used as a complement or supporting treatment for other medical conditions by relieving the musculoskeletal aspects associated with the condition. A recent Harvard Medical School review found that chiropractic care has expanded far beyond adjustments to include postural and exercise education, ergonomic training in walking and sitting to limit back strain, nutritional information, and some ultrasound therapies.

Chiropractic adjustment rarely causes discomfort and is safe when it's performed by someone who's trained and licensed to deliver chiropractic care. You may have mild soreness or aching following treatment, just as you would with some forms of exercise. But this soreness usually resolves within 12 to 48 hours after treatment.

Serious complications associated with chiropractic adjustment are rare but may include a herniated disk or compression of the nerves in your lower spinal column known as cauda equina syndrome, which can cause pain, weakness, loss of feeling in your legs and loss of bowel or bladder control. In very rare instances, it may cause a certain type of stroke known as vertebral artery dissection after neck manipulation.

Don't seek chiropractic adjustment if you have severe osteoporosis, numbness, tingling or loss of strength in an arm or leg, cancer in your spine, an increased risk of stroke, or an unstable spine. At your first visit, your chiropractor will ask questions about your health history and perform a physical exam, paying special attention to your spine. Your chiropractor may also recommend other examinations or tests, such as X-rays.

According to the American Chiropractic Association, chiropractic care can be traced all the way back to the beginning of recorded time. Writings from China and Greece from 2700 B.C. and 1500 B.C. mention spinal manipulation and how maneuvering the lower extremities helped ease low-back pain. The Greek physician Hippocrates, who lived from 460–357 B.C., also wrote about the importance of chiropractic care.

Although the roots of chiropractic care go way back in U.S. history, the practice of spinal manipulation didn't start catching on until the late 19th century.

In 1895, Daniel David Palmer founded the chiropractic profession in Davenport, Iowa. Palmer was well read in the medical journals of his time and had a lot of knowledge about developments in anatomy and physiology that were occurring throughout the world back then. He founded the Palmer School of Chiropractic in 1897, which is still one of the most prominent chiropractic colleges in the nation.

To receive a D.C., or Doctor of Chiropractic, degree, a person has to complete four to five years at an accredited chiropractic college. Chiropractors also have to pass a national board exam and any state tests before receiving a license to practice.

During a typical chiropractic adjustment, your chiropractor will place you in specific positions to treat affected areas. You'll often lie face down on a specially designed, padded chiropractic table. The chiropractor may use his or her hands to apply a controlled, sudden force to a joint, pushing it beyond its normal range of motion. You may hear popping or cracking sounds as your chiropractor moves your joints during the treatment session. Your chiropractor may recommend other types of treatment, too, such as heat or ice, massage, stretching, electrical stimulation, exercise or weight loss.

Some people experience minor side effects for a few days after chiropractic adjustment. These may include headache, fatigue or pain in the parts of the body that were treated. Not everyone responds to chiropractic adjustments. A lot depends on your particular situation. If your symptoms don't begin to improve after several weeks of treatments, chiropractic adjustment might not be the best option for you.

Most of the research done on spinal manipulation has focused on back pain, and many studies suggest that it does help. For example, a 2013 study in the Journal of Pain randomly assigned 110 adults with ages from 18–60 with chronic low-back pain to one of four treatment groups: actual spinal manipulation; a placebo consisting of a spinal manipulative sham procedure; an enhanced placebo—these people got the sham procedure and were told that it had been shown to significantly reduce low-back pain in some people; or no treatment at all.

For the spinal manipulation and sham treatments, a licensed physical therapist delivered six treatments over two weeks. The researchers found that spinal manipulation significantly reduced pain sensitivity when it was compared to the sham manipulation and no-treatment groups. But interestingly, the enhanced placebo was as effective a treatment as spinal manipulation—the people in this group were the most satisfied with their treatment.

Another study, this time a 2010 review of scientific evidence on manual therapies for a range of conditions, showed that spinal manipulation and mobilization may help treat several conditions in addition to back pain. Migraine and neck-related headaches, neck pain, upper- and lower-extremity joint conditions, and whiplash-associated disorders all made the list.

This review also identified a number of conditions that spinal manipulation or mobilization doesn't seem to help. These conditions included asthma, high blood pressure, and menstrual pain. For a number of symptoms and conditions, including fibromyalgia, mid-back pain, sciatica, and temporomandibular joint disorder, or TMJ, researchers couldn't say either way if treatment was helpful.

Researchers are continuing to study the safety of chiropractic treatment. A 2007 study of almost 20,000 people who received chiropractic treatment in the United Kingdom showed that minor side effects after cervical spine manipulation, such as temporary soreness, were relatively common, but that the risk of a serious adverse event was low or very low up to 7 days after treatment.

In an interview with The Chicago Tribune, Dr. Ralph Gay, vice chair of the Midwest Spine Care Practice within Mayo Clinic's Department of Physical Medicine and Rehabilitation, addressed the idea of safety within a larger conversation about how medical doctors view the field of chiropractic care. In his interview, Dr. Gay said that medical doctors generally have three main concerns about chiropractic care.

First, some medical doctors feel that the education requirements for chiropractors aren't rigorous enough. Unlike traditional medicine, there's no requirement for an internship or residency before a chiropractor is licensed.

Second, chiropractors don't police themselves very well. State boards regulate practice in all 50 states, but most chiropractors have their own private practice. That means that there's not much oversight, and there's not much reason for chiropractors to change the way they practice, even if there are changes they should make.

And finally, even if more sessions aren't needed, there's concern that chiropractors keep asking their patients to return. In general, the chiropractic practice model suggests that several treatments over a period of weeks or months is needed to get the most benefit. A trial period is usually 6–8 visits.

But these same concerns could be applied to physical therapy, acupuncture, and massage therapy. Although some chiropractors may look to their business models—more than they do clinical evidence—when they're deciding on a patient's treatment, most chiropractors limit treatment to what's needed for each individual patient based on their response to care.

Despite these concerns, Dr. Gay said in his interview that he sees medical doctors slowly changing their view of chiropractic care. They're not necessarily referring patients to chiropractors because they have a degree in chiropractic care; they're referring them in circumstances they feel such care could be helpful—and when they personally trust that a specific chiropractor will take good care of the patient.

In terms of chiropractic care, there are things you can do as a consumer to make sure you're getting the right kind and amount of care. In his interview, Dr. Gay suggests watching out for chiropractors who recommend initial treatment that lasts more than 3–4 weeks, who ask for lump-sum payment, or who want to treat you for a condition that's not related to the spine, or other common joint or muscle conditions.

If you're thinking about seeking chiropractic care, ask about the chiropractor's education and licensure. Bring up any medical conditions you have. Ask whether chiropractors have specialized training or experience in the condition you're looking for them to treat. Ask how much you'll be expected to pay and if insurance covers your treatment. Chiropractic adjustments are covered by many health maintenance organizations and private health plans, as well as Medicare, and state workers' compensation systems. Tell the chiropractor about any medications, prescription or over-the-counter, and dietary supplements you take. If a chiropractor suggests a dietary supplement, ask about potential interactions with your medications or other supplements.

Massage and spinal manipulation are not cures for diseases like cancer, heart disease, HIV or diabetes. However, massage has been shown to help manage pain, stress and anxiety that often accompany serious illness, surgery, and medical treatment. And both massage and spinal manipulation may help ease chronic muscle and joint pain, and can help you rebound from a sports injury. Massage is a pretty good remedy for the stresses and strains of daily life as well. Many healthy people use a weekly massage as a lifeline of peace and sanity in a busy and hectic world.

A spa is a fine place to get a massage and a place to try aromatherapy too. How could a spa visit improve your health? Join us next time and see.

Lecture 12

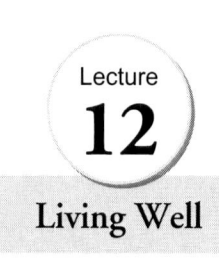

Living Well

From eating the right foods and exercising regularly to meditating and even spending time at a spa, every effort you make to improve your overall physical and mental health helps not just you, but also your family and even your community. In this lecture, you will learn how wellness centers and spa experiences may fit into your overall health and wellness program, and you will discover how happiness can positively affect your health.

Mayo Clinic's Healthy Living Program

- The Healthy Living Program at Mayo Clinic started with some observations by a longtime Mayo Clinic patient, Dan Abraham. In his visits to the clinic, he noticed that some of the Mayo Clinic staff looked stressed and unhealthy, and he wanted to do something about it.

- Over the years, through Dan Abraham's generosity, Mayo Clinic has been able to open a wellness center on its Rochester campus for employees and their families. The center was recently expanded to offer a wellness experience for Mayo Clinic patients and their families.

- A true wellness center, the Healthy Living Program brings together different areas—nutrition, fitness, and resiliency—along with spa activities, to help people feel better about themselves, improve their quality of life, and meet their goals with a comprehensive wellness plan that's unique to each individual.

- After visiting the Healthy Living Program, patients can go home and incorporate the tools and techniques they've learned into their lives, just as Mayo Clinic employees do when they visit the Healthy Living Center.

Aromatherapy

- Massage therapy is an important service of most spas, and it's often used with aromatherapy. The idea of aromatherapy is that certain scents can affect our psychological or physical well-being.

- Many people think that aromatherapy is about imagining a smell that makes us feel good, because scent is so connected to memory. That's certainly part of it. But another side to the practice of aromatherapy is focused on the therapeutic use of essential oils extracted from plants.

- Essential oils are concentrated extracts taken from the roots, leaves, seeds, or blossoms of plants. Each essential oil contains its own mix of active ingredients, and this mix determines what the oil is used for. Some oils are used to promote physical healing.

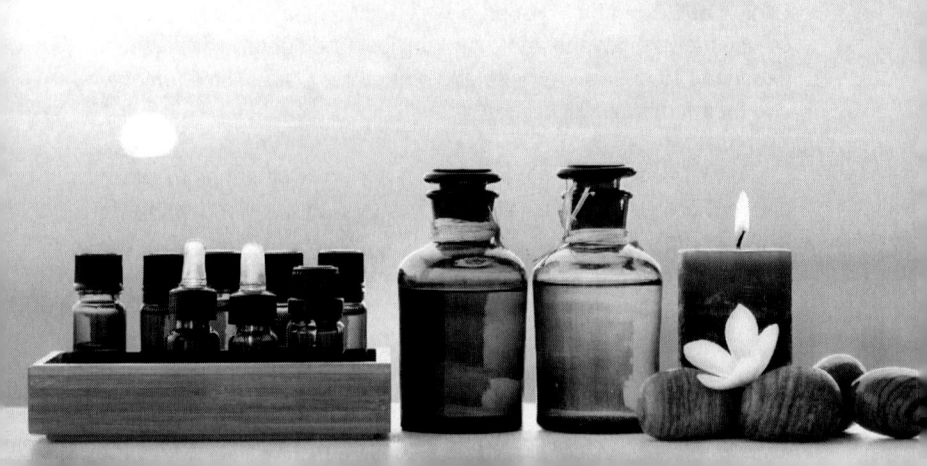

- Other plant oils can help you relax or make a room smell pleasant. Orange blossom oil or lavender oil, for example, contain a large amount of an active ingredient that's thought to be calming. The highly concentrated oils may be inhaled directly or indirectly, or applied to the skin through massage, lotions, or bath salts.

- Essential oils used in aromatherapy aren't regulated by the Food and Drug Administration, but for the most part, they're considered safe. However, just because they're natural doesn't mean that they don't pose risks if they're used inappropriately. It can be harmful to overuse or ingest essential oils, and they may produce some side effects or interactions.

- With aromatherapy massage, the idea is that your skin is able to absorb the essential oils at the sane time you're breathing in their scent and while you're experiencing the physical benefits of the massage. Common aromatherapy scents used for relaxation include lavender, jasmine, chamomile, bergamot, rose, sandalwood, and vanilla.

- Although there have been few formal studies of aromatherapy on humans, those that have been done suggest that aromatherapy may offer a number of health benefits. Some studies have shown aromatherapy can help relieve anxiety and symptoms of depression and improve quality of life, especially for people who have chronic health conditions.

Hot Tubs and Warm Pools

- Hot tubs provide another common spa experience. You can find hot tubs at pools, spas, and hotels. The hot water feels good and relaxes your muscles, lowers your blood pressure, and eases tension.

- Mayo Clinic researchers have found that soaking in a hot tub offers benefits similar to those from exercise, with less stress on the heart. Soaking in a hot tub increases your heart rate while lowering your blood pressure.

- Hot tubs aren't for everyone. Don't use a hot tub if you have any sort of wound, have severe respiratory problems, or are pregnant. In addition, hot tubs can be a breeding ground for dozens of types of bacteria, many of them potential pathogens. The water can be a ground zero for infectious diseases.

- There are many good reasons to approach hot tubs with caution, and for some people, they may make a calm, warm pool or a hot bath better options. Arthritis experts promote the use of warm-water pools as a way to reduce the force of gravity that's compressing a joint, support sore limbs, decrease swelling and inflammation, and increase circulation—all in just 20 minutes.

- Warm water helps by stimulating blood flow to stiff muscles and frozen joints. This makes a warm tub or pool a great place to do some gentle stretching. The flexibility lasts even after you get out.

- Warm water can be helpful in fighting the pain and stiffness of arthritis and fibromyalgia. A variety of studies show that people with both of these conditions who take part in warm-water exercise programs two or three times a week often are able to move more easily and experience significantly less pain. The exercise programs also provided an emotional boost, helped people sleep better, and were particularly effective for people who are overweight.

Saunas

- Saunas offer the opportunity to feel better through heat and sweat. Thomas Allison, Ph.D., director of Sports Cardiology at Mayo Clinic, says that there's no hard data to suggest that the use of saunas has any bearing on your overall health. Saunas can relax your muscles and make you feel good, but you should use them in moderation.

- Infrared saunas, sometimes called far-infrared saunas, use light to create heat. A traditional sauna uses heat to warm the air, which in turn warms your body. An infrared sauna heats your body directly without warming the air around you.

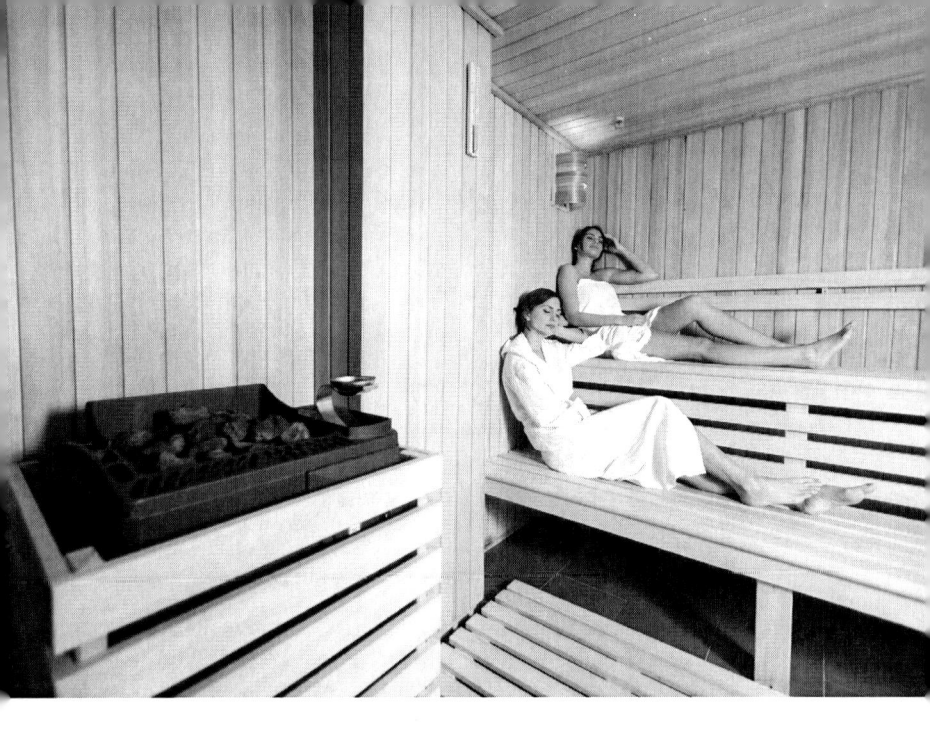

- The appeal of saunas in general is that they cause reactions, such as vigorous sweating and increased heart rate, similar to those elicited by moderate exercise. An infrared sauna produces these same results at lower temperatures than does a regular sauna, which makes it good for people who can't tolerate the heat of a conventional sauna.

- Several studies have looked at using infrared saunas to treat chronic health problems such as high blood pressure, congestive heart failure, and rheumatoid arthritis and found some evidence of benefit. However, larger and more rigorous studies are needed to confirm these results.

- On the other hand, no adverse effects have been reported with infrared saunas. So, if you're considering trying a sauna for relaxation, an infrared sauna might be an option.

- There's a lot more to many spas. They may also offer body treatments such as scrubs and wraps that are applied by massage therapists, as well as more conventional beauty treatments, such as facials, manicures, and pedicures.

- As with any complementary treatment, it's important to remember that nothing is without risk. Some cosmetic treatments can be dangerous if not carried out properly. You should never undergo any kind of spa treatment if you have an open cut or wound—that's how bacteria get in.

- Pay attention to how the spa cleans its equipment. Spas should use new or sanitized instruments on your hands and feet. See if they have an autoclave or sanitizing liquid, at the very least. If you see the technicians using the same files and clippers on each person, that's a sign that they aren't very clean, and you're taking a risk of getting an infection.

Spa Treatments

- A true, comprehensive spa can provide elements of wellness that go beyond the concept of pampering. And even if your doctor recognizes the importance of NESS (nutrition, exercise, stress management, and social support), he or she may not have the resources in his or her office to teach you tai chi or offer a massage. So, finding providers of these services in your own community is key—and so much the better if they have a working relationship with your health-care team.

- When you're looking for a great spa, look for a focus on stress management via massage or meditation training, aromatherapy, or yoga, as well as exercise opportunities and healthy eating.

- Think of the time spent in spa treatments as an investment in your health, not simple pampering. Even something as simple as a manicure or pedicure can be part of a wellness program.

- What you want from a "destination spa" may be different from what you need in your everyday wellness routine. Mayo Clinic's Healthy Living Center offers programs that Mayo Clinic employees and their families can participate in on an ongoing basis year-round, such as weight management, resiliency training, or thriving as a cancer survivor.

- But Mayo Clinic's Healthy Living Program is designed for people who are able to be there only for a short time. If you're thinking of participating in a destination spa program, look for one that will teach you what you need to know to continue with your program once you get home.

- You may be lucky enough to find a comprehensive wellness center in your community that offers massage, meditation training, maybe acupuncture, some nutrition coaching—all the things you have learned about in this course. Look for a place that can teach you some self-care skills, and maybe a place where you go once or twice a week for a massage or a class. In some areas, you may need to put together your program à la carte.

- Most massage and other spa treatments are not covered by insurance. Some are covered by health savings accounts, and many people are willing to pay for the treatments themselves, which speaks to how helpful they find them. When thinking about the cost of a yoga class or a massage, evaluate it against what you are willing to pay for coffee at a chain store.

Happiness and Health
- By increasing your level of happiness, you can improve your health and overall well-being. It's a big part of living well. The services you experience in a spa are designed to help you feel good, which

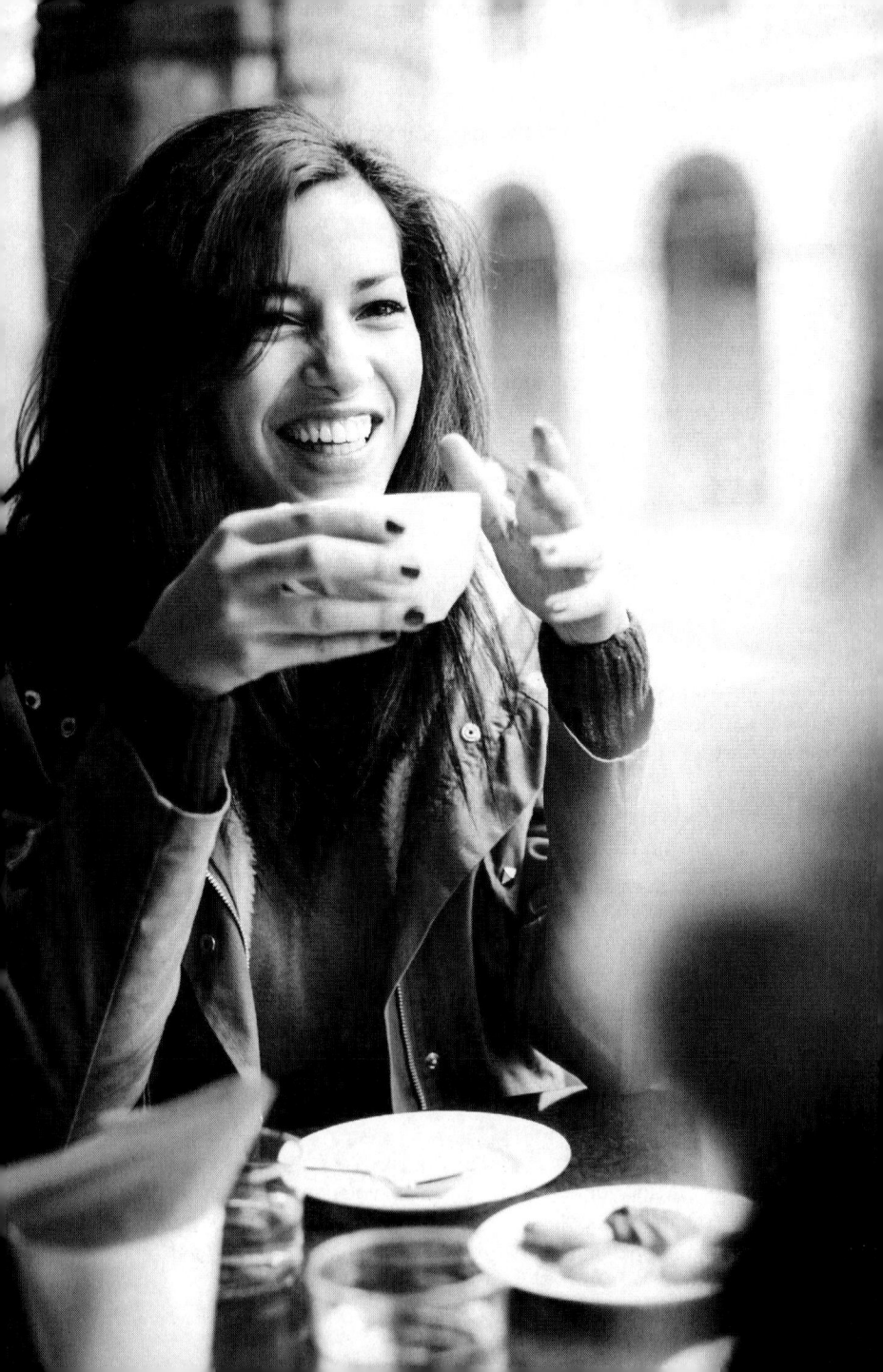

is certainly something that can help boost your happiness, but happiness means much more than that.

- Research shows that people who have a positive outlook on life do better in the long run than do those who see things negatively. In fact, a Mayo Clinic study found that optimists live about 20 percent longer than do pessimists.

- Changing your attitude can have direct effects on your health. By seeing life in a positive light, your health may benefit in many ways.

    - You may be less likely to be depressed.

    - You may have lower levels of distress.

    - You may be less likely to get the common cold.

    - You may have better psychological and physical well-being.

    - You may have a lower risk of death from cardiovascular disease.

    - You may be better able to cope with hardships and stress.

- It's not completely clear why people who have a positive outlook on life experience these health benefits. One theory is that a positive attitude enables you to cope better with stressful situations, reducing the harmful health effects of stress on your body. It's also thought that positive and optimistic people tend to live healthier lifestyles; they get more physical activity, follow a healthier diet, and don't smoke or drink alcohol in excess.

- Like stress, negative self-talk can also have harmful effects on your health. That's bad news if you naturally tend to feel depressed. But the good news is that this seems to be a personality trait that you can change with practice. For many people, that means putting a stop to the negative messages they mentally tell themselves. Constantly reinforcing those negative messages just increases the chances that you won't succeed.

- Look at the areas of your life you want to change and start small by identifying incremental changes you can make to get yourself moving in the right direction. Surround yourself with positive people who will help provide encouragement rather than undermine you or make you doubt yourself and your ability to achieve your goals.

- It may take a bit of practice to get into the habit of more positive self-talk. Try to not say anything to yourself that you wouldn't say to anyone else. Most people tend to be their own harshest critics. At the same time, don't forget your NESS program. Eat a healthy diet and exercise regularly to positively affect your mood and reduce stress.

Suggested Reading

Allison, et al, "Cardiovascular Responses to Immersion in a Hot Tub."

Buettner, *The Blue Zones.*

Maruta, et al, "Optimism-Pessimism Assessed in the 1960s."

Maruta, et al, "Optimists vs. Pessimists."

Texas A&M University, "A Risky Soaking."

Lecture 12 Transcript

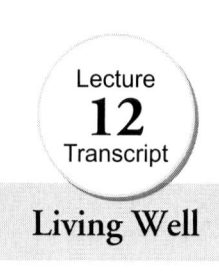

Living Well

If there's one thing I hope you take away from this course, it's that it is possible for you to put together an integrative program that can positively affect your health. In this lecture, I'd like to talk about how and why we created Mayo Clinic's Healthy Living Program and ways that you can bring these concepts into your own life and into your community.

The Healthy Living Program at Mayo Clinic actually started with some observations by a longtime Mayo Clinic patient, Dan Abraham. In his visits to the clinic, he noticed that some of the Mayo Clinic staff looked stressed and unhealthy, and he wanted to do something about it. Over the years, through Dan Abraham's generosity, Mayo Clinic has been able to open a wellness center on its Rochester campus for employees and their families. We recently expanded the center by adding two more floors, this time to offer a wellness experience for Mayo Clinic patients and their families.

A true wellness center, the Healthy Living Program brings together different areas—nutrition, fitness, and resiliency—along with spa activities, to help people feel better about themselves, improve their quality of life and meet their goals with a comprehensive wellness plan that's unique to each individual.

After visiting the Healthy Living Program, patients can go home and incorporate the tools and techniques they've learned into their lives, just as Mayo Clinic employees do when they visit the Healthy Living Center.

You may have noticed that in my description of what the Healthy Living Program offers, I said spa. The term spa has been somewhat corrupted in modern usage. It originally meant a health resort, a place where you would take to the waters, eat right and get some exercise in the fresh air. Today, you see the word spa used for everything from a nail spa to a dog spa. But if we stick with the historical definition of a spa—a place that promotes health and healing—then incorporating spa into everything else we're doing at Mayo Clinic makes perfect sense.

As medical director of Rejuvenate Spa at the Healthy Living Program, I had already done plenty of research on massage, meditation, acupuncture and other complementary approaches. So those made perfect sense to me to be included as part of an overall wellness approach. But I have to admit, I was a bit skeptical when the idea of including any kind of beauty services was brought up because I wanted people to understand that the services we provided were about more than beauty. Eventually, I came to realize that looking better made patients feel better. And sometimes, they needed to see that little bit of change—they needed to feel just a little bit better about themselves—before they were ready to take on some of the next steps in their wellness journeys. And of course, once I was finally brave enough to go and experience a facial, I had a new respect for the power of what some of these aesthetic services can provide.

My first interest is helping patients to understand how a spa fits into an overall wellness program, and that incorporating routine spa services into their program isn't about pampering—it's about using evidence-based therapies to help promote health and wellness on an ongoing basis. But I also quickly learned that a spa can be a place to help address immediate needs, too.

Patients and their families are often at Mayo Clinic for three to five days of what can be grueling tests, experiments, and treatment. Many are struggling with life-defining illnesses, so stress can be high—for the patients and for their loved ones. And if you remember our earlier discussions, stress can suppress our immune function or slow how quickly wounds heal—exactly what we don't want to see happen to our patients when they're being treated for cancer or undergoing surgery.

With all of this said, I'm finding that when they come to Mayo Clinic for care, more and more of my patients are booking time in between their appointments to get a massage or take a yoga class in the spa. And since caregivers experience almost as much stress as their loved ones do, when someone is going through treatment, many spouses and significant others are spending time in the steam room while their loved one is in the midst of a lengthy test or procedure. We're starting to see more people who recognize that dealing with stress—whether it's acute or chronic—is important, and that spa treatments can be a perfect adjunct to healthy nutrition and exercise to help manage stress.

You may be wondering, Where did you develop your interest in spa services? I've served on the foundation board of the International Spa Association for several years and am currently the medical advisor for all of ISPA. During the time I've been involved in the ISPA, I've had a firsthand view as spas have moved from being seen as places of pampering to key components of individual wellness strategies. I've become very convinced that there's a great opportunity for spa services and medicine to complement each other in the health and wellness arena. That's why I was enthusiastic about offering massage therapy from the outset, for example. I had seen the benefit it could provide patients who were undergoing a variety of treatments—from surgery to chemotherapy—and I could see how much it helped our staff as well.

So let's look into spa services and what they include. Massage therapy, which you learned about earlier in this course, is an important service of most spas, and it's often used with aromatherapy. The idea of aromatherapy is that certain scents can affect our psychological or physical wellbeing. A lot of people think that aromatherapy is about imagining a smell that makes us feel good because scent is so connected to memory. That's certainly part of it—maybe the smell of apples baking in a pie makes you feel happy and relaxed.

But another side to the practice of aromatherapy is focused on the therapeutic use of essential oils extracted from plants. Essential oils are concentrated extracts taken from the roots, leaves, seeds or blossoms of plants. Each essential oil contains its own mix of active ingredients, and this mix determines what the oil is used for. Some oils are used to promote physical healing, for example, to treat swelling or fungal infections.

Other plant oils can help you relax or make a room smell pleasant. Orange blossom oil or lavender oil, for example, contain a large amount of an active ingredient that's thought to be calming. The highly concentrated oils may be inhaled directly or indirectly, or applied to the skin through massage, lotions or bath salts.

This is nothing new. Essential oils have been used for therapeutic purposes for thousands of years—by Chinese, Indian, Egyptian, Greek and Roman civilizations, among others. Our modern term aromatherapy was coined in 1927, by French chemist René-Maurice Gattefossé. He discovered the healing properties of lavender oil when he applied it to a burn on his hand caused by an explosion in his laboratory. That accident inspired him to analyze the chemical properties of essential oils and later study how they could be used to treat burns, skin infections, gangrene, and wounds experienced by soldiers during World War I.

Essential oils used in aromatherapy aren't regulated by the Food and Drug Administration, but for the most part, they're considered safe. However, just because they're natural doesn't mean that they don't pose risks if they're used inappropriately. It can be harmful to overuse or ingest essential oils, and they may produce some side effects or interactions. Inhaling essential oils isn't likely to be toxic, but you may be sensitive to an essential oil if you're in a non-ventilated room, the temperature is very high, and there is a constant diffusion of essential oil that saturates the air.

Essential oils are often applied to the skin, so it's important to know about adverse skin reactions they may cause. Essential oils can cause allergic reactions, skin irritation and sun sensitivity. There's not much evidence out there on the safety or efficacy of oils taken orally, so we generally stick to inhalation or topical use.

With aromatherapy massage, the idea is that your skin is able to absorb the essential oils at the same time you're breathing in their scent and while you're experiencing the physical benefits of the massage. Common aromatherapy scents used for relaxation include lavender, jasmine, chamomile, bergamot, rose, sandalwood and vanilla.

Although there have been few formal studies of aromatherapy on humans, those that have been done suggest that aromatherapy may offer a number of health benefits. Some studies have shown aromatherapy can help relieve anxiety and symptoms of depression and improve quality of life, especially for people who have chronic health conditions. Smaller studies suggest that aromatherapy with lavender oil may help make needle sticks less painful for people receiving dialysis, improve sleep for people who are hospitalized, and reduce pain for children undergoing tonsillectomy. When massage therapy is used in addition to medications or psychotherapy, the use of essential oils seems to help people with depression. The benefits seem to be related to relaxation caused by the scents and the massage.

Clinical studies involving qualified midwives showed that when the midwives used essential oils—in particular, rose, lavender, and frankincense—they were able to help pregnant women feel less anxiety and fear, have a stronger sense of well-being, and need less pain medication during delivery. Some women also say that peppermint oil helps relieve nausea and vomiting during labor.

At Mayo Clinic, we use aromatherapy in a variety of ways. For example, if a patient is nervous or anxious before a procedure, we may offer a sample of lavender that the patient can inhale to help ease anxiety and enhance overall relaxation. Spearmint and ginger may help manage nausea. Lavender samples may also be offered to help with sleeplessness and as a way to help manage pain. Essential oils may also be used with other Integrative Medicine services, such as massage, acupuncture or stress management counseling.

Hot tubs provide another common spa experience—you can find hot tubs at pools, spas and hotels. The hot water feels good and relaxes your muscles, lowers your blood pressure and eases tension.

Mayo Clinic researchers have found that soaking in a hot tub offers benefits similar to those from exercise, with less stress on the heart. Soaking in a hot tub increases your heart rate while lowering your blood pressure. We used to worry that hot tubs weren't safe for people with heart conditions, but one study looked at 15 men with stable coronary artery disease and found no problems in a typical 15-minute soak in 104-degree water. With that said, hot tubs aren't for everyone. Don't use a hot tub if you have any sort of wound, have severe respiratory problems, or are pregnant.

In addition, hot tubs can be a breeding ground for dozens of types of bacteria, many of them potential pathogens. The water can be ground zero for infectious diseases.

In a recent study, Texas A&M microbiologist Dr. Rita B. Moyes tested 43 water samples from whirlpool bathtubs—both private and public ones—and found that all 43 had bacterial growth ranging from mild to dangerous. Almost all of them showed the presence of fecal-derived bacteria while more than three-quarters of them had fungi and more than a third of them contained *staphylococcus*, which can cause deadly staph infections.

In this research, Dr. Moyes added that such harmful bacteria can lead to numerous diseases, such as urinary tract infections, septicemia, pneumonia and several types of skin infections. She explained that the aerosol mist created by the whirlpool action forces microbes into the lungs or open cuts.

At Mayo Clinic, we diagnosed a condition called hot tub lung, where people had coughing, shortness of breath and fever, all from bacteria that they inhaled from a hot tub. Some of their oxygen levels dropped to such dangerous levels that they had to be put on oxygen.

These are all good reasons to approach hot tubs with caution, and for some of you, they may make a calm, warm pool or a hot bath better options. Arthritis experts promote the use of warm water pools as a way to reduce the force of gravity that's compressing a joint, support sore limbs, decrease swelling and inflammation, and increase circulation—all in just 20 minutes.

Warm water helps by stimulating blood flow to stiff muscles and frozen joints. This makes a warm tub or pool a great place to do some gentle stretching. The flexibility lasts even after you get out.

Warm water can be so helpful in fighting the pain and stiffness of arthritis and fibromyalgia. A variety of studies show that people with both of these conditions who take part in warm-water exercise program two or three times a week often are able to move more easily and experience significantly less pain. The exercise programs also provided an emotional boost, helped people sleep better, and were particularly effective for people who are overweight.

The use of saunas goes back centuries. Today, native Americans still use sweat lodges; the Finnish have saunas; the Russians banyas. They all offer the opportunity to feel better through heat and sweat. Dr. Thomas Allison, director of Sports Cardiology at Mayo Clinic, says there's no hard data to suggest that the use of saunas has any bearing on your overall health. Saunas can relax your muscles and make you feel good, but you should use them in moderation.

Here at Mayo Clinic, we've looked at infrared saunas, which use light to create heat. These saunas are sometimes called far-infrared saunas—far describes where the infrared waves fall on the light spectrum. A traditional sauna uses heat to warm the air, which in turn warms your body. An infrared sauna heats your body directly without warming the air around you.

The appeal of saunas, in general, is that they cause reactions, such as vigorous sweating and increased heart rate, similar to those elicited by moderate exercise. An infrared sauna produces these same results at lower temperatures than does a regular sauna, which makes it good for people who can't tolerate the heat of a conventional sauna. But does that translate into tangible health benefits? Perhaps.

Several studies have looked at using infrared saunas to treat chronic health problems such as high blood pressure, congestive heart failure and rheumatoid arthritis, and found some evidence of benefit. However, larger and more rigorous studies are needed to confirm these results. On the other hand, no adverse effects have been reported with infrared saunas. So if you're considering trying a sauna for relaxation, an infrared sauna might be an option.

There's a lot more to many spas. They may also offer body treatments such as scrubs and wraps that are applied by massage therapists, as well as more conventional beauty treatments like facials, manicures, and pedicures.

As with any complementary treatment, it's important to remember that nothing is without risk. Some cosmetic treatments that can be dangerous if not carried out properly. You should never undergo any kind of spa treatment if you have an open cut or wound—that's how bacteria get in. Pay attention to how the spa cleans its equipment. Spas should use new or sanitized instruments on your hands and feet—see if they have an autoclave or sanitizing liquid at the very least.

If you see the technicians using the same files and clippers on each person, that's a sign they aren't very clean, and you're taking a risk of getting an infection. In the Rejuvenate Spa at the Mayo Clinic Healthy Living Program, we put a lot of effort into redesigning every aspect of each treatment to minimize the risk of infection. We insist on applying Mayo Clinic standards of cleanliness and sterility to the spa setting, and that's something you should look for, too.

A true, comprehensive spa can provide elements of wellness that go beyond the concept of pampering. And even if your doctor recognizes the importance of N.E.S.S., he or she may not have the resources in his or her office to teach you tai chi or offer a massage. So finding providers of these services in your own community is key—and so much the better if they have a working relationship with your health-care team.

Before we opened Rejuvenate Spa, I visited a number of the massage therapy locations and acupuncture practices in town so that if I wanted one of my patients to experience these treatments, I knew what to expect from the providers. The providers communicated to me observations they had regarding the patient, and the patient received a uniform message from everyone involved in his or her care. This is the ideal situation in terms of integrating all of the care you receive.

Rejuvenate Spa is a natural outgrowth of Mayo Clinic's recognition of the value of these services, and the importance of having them occur in collaboration with the best of conventional care. That's why we brought all of these types of care under one roof.

So when you're looking for a great spa, keep the idea behind Rejuvenate Spa in mind. Look for a focus similar to what we've talked about in this course—stress management via massage or meditation, aromatherapy, yoga, as well as exercise opportunities and healthy eating. Think of the time spent in spa treatments as an investment in your health, not simple pampering. Even something as simple as a manicure or pedicure can be part of a wellness program. I've had many patients at Rejuvenate, who came in for manicures but signed up for our yoga or nutrition class on the way out the door.

What you want from a destination spa may be different from what you need in your everyday wellness routine. Mayo Clinic's Healthy Living Center offers programs that Mayo Clinic employees and their families can participate in on an ongoing basis year-round, such as weight management, resiliency training, or thriving as a cancer survivor.

But, as I mentioned at the beginning of this lecture, Mayo Clinic's Healthy Living Program is designed for people who are able to be here only for a short time. If you're thinking of participating in a destination spa program, look for one that will teach you what you need to know to continue with your program once you get home.

You may be lucky enough to find a comprehensive wellness center in your own community that offers massage, meditation training, maybe acupuncture, some nutrition coaching—all the things we've talked about in this course. Look for a place that can teach you some self-care skills, and maybe a place where you go once or twice a week for a massage or a class. In some areas, you may need to put together your program a la carte.

Most massage and other spa treatments are not covered by insurance. Some are covered by health savings accounts, and many people are willing to pay for the treatments themselves, which speaks to how helpful they find them. When thinking about the cost of a yoga class or a massage, you should evaluate it against what you are willing to pay for coffee at a chain store.

Now that you've learned a little bit about how wellness centers and spa experiences may fit into your overall health and wellness program, I'd like to tie everything we've learned in this course together with a discussion about a very important topic: the relationship that happiness has to your health. By increasing your level of happiness, you can improve your health and your overall well-being. It's a big part of living well. I mentioned in our discussion of spa services that the services you experience in a spa are designed to help you feel good—that's certainly something that can help boost your happiness. But happiness means much more than that.

Let's start our discussion about happiness by delving into the power of positive thinking.

Research shows that people who have a positive outlook on life do better in the long run than do those who see things negatively. As a matter of fact, one Mayo Clinic study found that optimists live about 20% longer than do pessimists. On the surface, you might think that's simply due to their underlying health—it's not hard to believe that people who are healthy might just naturally feel happier. But controlled studies suggest that the situation works the other way around, too. Changing your attitude can have direct effects on your health. By seeing life in a positive light, your health may benefit in many ways. You may be less likely to be depressed; you may have lower levels of distress; you may be less likely to get the common cold; you may have better psychological and physical well-being; you may have a lower risk of death from cardiovascular disease; you may be better able to cope with hardships and stress.

It's not completely clear why people who have a positive outlook on life experience these health benefits. One theory is that a positive attitude enables you to cope better with stressful situations, which reduces the harmful health effects of stress on your body. It's also thought that positive and optimistic people tend to live healthier lifestyles—they get more physical activity, follow a healthier diet, and don't smoke or drink alcohol in excess.

And if you think back to some of the negative effects of stress we've discussed earlier in this course, it's not too hard to see why having a positive outlook on life can have the opposite effect of stress—and can lead to better health.

Like stress, negative self-talk can also have harmful effects on your health. That's bad news if you naturally tend to feel depressed. But the good news is that this seems to be a personality trait that you can change with practice. For a lot of people, that means putting a stop to the negative messages they mentally tell themselves. I have a lot of patients who, when they come in to see me, preface their concerns with, "I've tried everything, but I just can't exercise," or, "I tried to lose weight, but nothing works for me." Constantly reinforcing those negative messages just increases the chances that you won't succeed.

So, first off, stop telling yourself that you can't do something. Look at the areas of your life you want to change—maybe it's your weight, maybe it's your blood pressure, maybe it's your ability to keep up with your grandchildren on the playground—and start small by identifying incremental changes you can make to get yourself moving in the right direction. If you find negative thoughts creeping into your mind like, "I'm never going to lose weight," redirect your thoughts to something you can do right away, like taking a short walk around the block or even taking three deep breaths. From there, surround yourself with positive people who will help provide encouragement rather than undermine you or make you doubt yourself and your ability to achieve your goals.

It may take a bit of practice to get into the habit of more positive self-talk. One simple rule we suggest at Mayo Clinic is this: Don't say anything to yourself that you wouldn't say to anyone else. Try it. Most of us tend to be our own harshest critics, and that's usually not helpful. And at the same time, don't forget your N.E.S.S. program. Eat a healthy diet and exercise regularly to positively affect your mood and reduce stress.

Before we end our course, I want to return to our theme of integrative medicine. We've talked about some ancient practices, like traditional Chinese medicine and yoga, but I want to let you in on some cutting-edge practices as well. Some of the most exciting things I've seen are taking place in our Well Living Lab, a collaborative effort between Mayo Clinic and Delos, a company that specializes in what's called wellness real estate. They focus on transforming homes, offices, schools and other indoor environments into places that focus on health and wellness. Amenities included in their building designs come from research-supported suggestions for improving an individual's wellbeing.

Delos observed that 90% of our time is spent indoors, so they look at factors like building standards, acoustics, lighting and air quality and how these amenities can be shaped to enhance personal wellness. The Well Living Lab simulates realistic living and working environments, like schools, offices and hotels, to monitor how well the health-based interventions work.

In the 6,000-square-foot Well Living Lab, sensors measure how people react to changes in their environment. Here's a good example of one of the sensors: There's a chair that buzzes when your butt's been in it too long. That's important, now that we know that prolonged sitting is bad for your health—and we've learned that even long hours at the gym don't seem to offset the risk of sitting too much can have on your health. Sensors like this one at the Well Living Lab illustrate one way we can modify the environments we operate in to promote health and wellness and help us live healthier lives.

The point with the Well Living Lab—and really, everything we've talked about in this course—is that it's crucial that you play an active role in your health and well-being. Part of taking responsibility involves looking around at your environment and giving some thought to tools that can help you, and even your community, be healthier and happier.

Research conducted by Dan Buettner, working with National Geographic and a team of scientists and organizations that specialize in aging, found that people in certain areas of the world tend to live longer, healthier, happier lives and experience very few of the diseases that affect others. In these areas of the world, called Blue Zones, people are three times more likely than most Americans to live to be 100 years old—and still enjoy life.

Researchers, anthropologists, demographers and epidemiologists involved in the Blue Zones project find clear and common reasons why these people lived longer, healthier, happier lives, and those reasons probably won't surprise you. They're exactly the opposite of the trends I outlined at the beginning of this course: people in the Blue Zones stay in motion throughout the day, have a sense of purpose, use stress management techniques, eat moderately and eat very little red meat, and are involved with their families and their communities.

And here's a really interesting note about the Blue Zones: People who lived the longest were part of social networks that included other people who lived long lives—people whose healthy behaviors seemed to rub off on them. This makes sense and shouldn't surprise us. Research shows that smoking, obesity, and even loneliness are contagious. So why not create some behaviors you'd want to spread?

Take a moment and really think about this. Think about the things you can do each day to improve your wellness—think N.E.S.S—nutrition, exercise, stress management, and support. What do you do each day to support your wellness in these areas? From eating the right foods and exercising regularly to meditating and even spending time at a spa, every effort you make to improve your overall physical and mental health helps not just you, but also your family and even your community. Healthy habits have a powerful ripple effect. So look around every day to see what you can do to support your own personal wellness and help others in your community lead healthier, happier lives.

You can do it.

Bibliography

Allison, Thomas G., et al. "Cardiovascular Responses to Immersion in a Hot Tub in Comparison with Exercise in Male Subjects with Coronary Artery Disease." *Mayo Clinic Proceedings* 68, no. 1 (1993): 19–25.

Balasubramaniam, Meera, et al. "Yoga on Our Minds: A Systematic Review of Yoga for Neuropsychiatric Disorders." *Frontiers in Psychiatry* 3, no. 117 (2013): 1–16.

Bardia, Aditya, et al. "Efficacy of Complementary and Alternative Medicine Therapies in Relieving Cancer Pain: A Systematic Review." *Journal of Clinical Oncology* 24, no. 34 (2006): 5457–5464.

Barton, Debra L., et al. "Pilot Study of Panax Quinquefolius (American Ginseng) to Improve Cancer-Related Fatigue: A Randomized, Double-Blind, Dose-Finding Evaluation: NCCTG Trial N03CA." *Supportive Care in Cancer* 18, no. 2 (2010): 179–187.

Barton, Debra L., et al. "The Use of Valeriana Officinalis (Valerian) in Improving Sleep in Patients Who Are Undergoing Treatment for Cancer: A Phase III Randomized, Placebo-Controlled, Double-Blind Study: NCCTG Trial, N01C5." *Journal of Supportive Oncology* 9, no. 1 (2011): 24–31.

Bauer, Brent A. "Chinese Medicine and Integrative Medicine in the United States." *Chinese Journal of Integrative Medicine* 21, no. 8 (2015): 569–70.

Bauer, Brent A., et al. "Effect of Massage Therapy on Pain, Anxiety, and Tension after Cardiac Surgery: A Randomized Study." *Complementary Therapies in Clinical Practice* 16, no. 2 (2010): 70–75.

Bauer, Brent A., et al. "Effect of the Combination of Music and Nature Sounds on Pain and Anxiety in Cardiac Surgical Patients: A Randomized Study." *Alternative Therapies in Health and Medicine* 17, no. 4 (2011): 16–23.

Bauer, Brent A., medical ed. *Mayo Clinic Book of Alternative Medicine*. 2nd ed. Rochester, MN: Mayo Foundation for Medical Education and Research, 2010.

Bays, Jan Chozen. *How to Train a Wild Elephant: And Other Adventures in Mindfulness*. Boston: Shambhala Publications, 2011.

Bronfort, Gert, et al. "Effectiveness of Manual Therapies: The UK Evidence Report." *Chiropractic & Osteopathy* 18 (2010): 1–33.

Bruce, Barbara K., and Tracy E. Harrison, medical eds. *Mayo Clinic Guide to Pain Relief*. Rochester, MN: Mayo Foundation for Medical Education and Research, 2013.

Buenz, E. J., et al. "Bioprospecting Rumphius's Ambonese Herbal: Volume I." *Journal of Ethnopharmacology* 96, no. 1–2 (2005): 57–70.

Buettner, Dan. *The Blue Zones, Second Edition: 9 Lessons for Living Longer from the People Who've Lived the Longest*. Washington, DC: National Geographic Society, 2012.

Carlson, Jennifer R., et al. "Reading the Tea Leaves: Anticarcinogenic Properties of (-)-Epigallocatechin-3-Gallate." *Mayo Clinic Proceedings* 82, no. 6 (2007): 725–732.

Centers for Disease Control and Prevention. "Sleep and Sleep Disorders." http://www.cdc.gov/sleep/index.html. Accessed June 10, 2015.

Chan, Agnes S., et al. "A Chinese *Chan*-Based Mind-Body Intervention for Patients with Depression." *Journal of Affective Disorders* 142 (2012): 283–289.

Chan, Jessie S. M., et al. "Qigong Exercise Alleviates Fatigue, Anxiety, and Depressive Symptoms, Improves Sleep Quality, and Shortens Sleep Latency in Persons with Chronic Fatigue Syndrome-Like Illness." *Evidence-Based Complementary and Alternative Medicine* 2014 (2014): 1–10.

Chang-Miller, April, medical ed. *Mayo Clinic on Arthritis*. Rochester, MN: Mayo Foundation for Medical Education and Research, 2013.

Chesak, Sherry S., et al. "Enhancing Resilience among New Nurses: Feasibility and Efficacy of a Pilot Intervention." *The Ochsner Journal* 15, no. 1 (2015): 38–44.

Clair, Alicia Ann, et al. "A Feasibility Study of the Effects of Music and Movement on Physical Function, Quality of Life, Depression, and Anxiety in Patients with Parkinson Disease." *Music and Medicine* 4, no. 1 (2012): 49–55.

Clarke, Tainya C., et al. "Trends in the Use of Complementary Health Approaches among Adults: United States, 2002–2012." *National Health Statistics Report*. U.S. Department of Health and Human Services, Centers for Disease Control and Prevention, National Center for Health Statistics. February 10, 2015. http://www.cdc.gov/nchs/data/nhsr/nhsr079.pdf.

Clegg, Daniel O., et al. "Glucosamine, Chondroitin Sulfate, and the Two in Combination for Painful Knee Osteoarthritis." *New England Journal of Medicine* 254, no. 8 (2006): 795–808.

Coleman, Jane F. "Spring Forest Qigong and Chronic Pain." *Journal of Holistic Nursing* 29, no. 2 (2011): 118–128.

ConsumerLab.com. "How to Read a ConsumerLab.com Approved Quality Product Seal." http://www.consumerlab.com/seal.asp. Accessed February 2, 2016.

Creagan, Edward T., medical ed. *Mayo Clinic on Healthy Aging*. Rochester, MN: Mayo Foundation for Medical Education and Research, 2013.

Creagan, Edward T., et al. "Animal-Assisted Therapy at Mayo Clinic: The Time Is Now." *Complementary Therapies in Clinical Practice* 21, no. 2 (2015): 101–104.

Cutshall, Susanne M., et al. "A Decade of Offering a Healing Enhancement Program at an Academic Medical Center." *Complementary Therapies in Clinical Practice* 21, no. 4 (2015): 211–216.

Cutshall, Susanne M., et al. "Creation of a Healing Enhancement Program at an Academic Medical Center." *Complementary Therapies in Clinical Practice* 13, no. 4 (2007): 217–223.

Cutshall, Susanne M., et al. "Effect of Massage Therapy on Pain, Anxiety, and Tension in Cardiac Surgical Patients: A Pilot Study." *Complementary Therapies in Clinical Practice* 16, no. 2 (2010): 92–95.

Cutshall, Susanne M., et al. "Evaluation of a Biofeedback-Assisted Meditation Program as a Stress Management Tool for Hospital Nurses: A Pilot Study." *Explore (NY)* 7, no. 2 (2011): 110–112.

Cutshall, Susanne M., et al. "Symptom Burden and Integrative Medicine in Cancer Survivorship." *Supportive Care in Cancer* 23, no. 10 (2015): 2989–2994.

Dahm, Diane, and Jay Smith, editors in chief. *Mayo Clinic Fitness for EveryBody.* Rochester, MN: Mayo Foundation for Medical Education and Research, 2005.

Dasse, Michelle N., et al. "Hypnotizability, Not Suggestion, Influences False Memory Development." *International Journal of Clinical and Experimental Hypnosis* 63, no. 1 (2015): 110–128.

Deardorff, Julie. "A Medical Doctor's View of Chiropractic Care." *Chicago Tribune.* August 4, 2009. http://featuresblogs.chicagotribune.com/features_julieshealthclub/2009/08/a-medical-doctors-take-on-chiropractic-care.html.

DiFiore, Nancy. Rush University Medical Center. "Diet May Help Prevent Alzheimer's." https://www.rush.edu/print/1012076.

———. Rush University Medical Center. "New MIND Diet May Significantly Protect against Alzheimer's Disease." https://www.rush.edu/news/press-releases/new-mind-diet-may-significantly-protect-against-alzheimers-disease.

Dion, Liza J., et al. "Development of a Hospital-Based Massage Therapy Course at an Academic Medical Center." *International Journal of Therapeutic Massage & Bodywork* 8, no. 1 (2015): 25–30.

Dion, Liza J., et al. "Effect of Massage on Pain Management for Thoracic Surgery Patients." *International Journal of Therapeutic Massage & Bodywork* 4, no. 2 (2011): 2–6.

Dion, Liza J., et al. "Massage Therapy Alone and in Combination with Meditation for Breast Cancer Patients Undergoing Autologous Tissue Reconstruction: A Randomized Pilot Study." *Complementary Therapies in Clinical Practice* May 12 (2015) [Epub ahead of print].

Drackley, Nancy L., et al. "Effect of Massage Therapy for Postsurgical Mastectomy Recipients." *Clinical Journal of Oncology Nursing* 16, no. 2 (2012): 121–124.

Dreyer, Nikol E., et al. "Effect of Massage Therapy on Pain, Anxiety, Relaxation, and Tension after Colorectal Surgery: A Randomized Study." *Complementary Therapies in Clinical Practice* 21, no. 3 (2015): 154–159.

Edakkanambeth Varayil, J., et al. "Over-the-Counter Enzyme Supplements: What a Clinician Needs to Know." *Mayo Clinic Proceedings* 89, no. 9 (2014): 1307–1312.

Engen, Deborah J., et al. "Feasibility and Effect of Chair Massage Offered to Nurses during Work Hours on Stress-Related Symptoms: A Pilot Study." *Complementary Therapies in Clinical Practice* 18, no. 4 (2012): 212–215.

Engen, Deborah J., et al. "The Effect of Chair Massage on Muscular Discomfort in Cardiac Sonographers: A Pilot Study." *BMC Complementary and Alternative Medicine* 10, no. 50 (2010).

Flugel Colle, Kathleen F, et al. "Measurement of Quality of Life and Participant Experience with the Mindfulness-Based Stress Reduction Program." *Complementary Therapies in Clinical Practice* 16, no. 1 (2010): 36–40.

Foji, Samira, et al. "The Study of the Effect of Guided Imagery on Pain, Anxiety and Some Other Hemodynamic Factors in Patients Undergoing Coronary Angiography." *Complementary Therapies in Clinical Practice* 21, no. 2 (2015): 119–123.

Fong, Shirley S. M., et al. "The Effects of a 6-Month Tai Chi Qigong Training Program on Temporomandibular, Cervical, and Shoulder Joint Mobility and Sleep Problems in Nasopharyngeal Cancer Survivors." *Integrative Cancer Therapies* 14, no. 1 (2015): 16–25.

Gaik, Frances. "Qigong as an Alternative and Complementary Treatment for Depression: A Preliminary Study Applying Spring Forest Qigong to Depression as an Alternative & Complementary Treatment." Saarbrücken, Germany: LAP Lambert Academic Publishing AG & Co. KG, 2010.

"Get the Facts: Yoga for Health." National Center for Complementary and Alternative Medicine. https://nccih.nih.gov/health/yoga/introduction.htm. Accessed July 17, 2015.

Gonzales, Eric A., et al. "Effects of Guided Imagery on Postoperative Outcomes in Patients Undergoing Same-Day Surgical Procedures: A Randomized, Single-Blind Study." *AANA Journal* 78, no. 3 (2010): 181–188.

Goyal, Madhav, et al. "Meditation Programs for Psychological Stress and Wellbeing: A Systematic Review and Meta-Analysis." *JAMA Internal Medicine* 174, no. 3 (2014): 357–368.

Grogan, Martha, medical ed. *Mayo Clinic Healthy Heart for Life.* New York: Time Home Entertainment, Inc., 2012.

Guo, Ruoling, et al. "Hawthorn Extract for Treating Chronic Heart Failure (Review)." *Cochrane Database of Systematic Reviews* 11 (2013).

Habermann, Thomas M., et al. "Complementary and Alternative Medicine Use Among Long-Term Lymphoma Survivors: A Pilot Study." *American Journal of Hematology* 84, no. 12 (2009): 795–798.

Hagen, Philip, and Martha Millman, medical eds. *Mayo Clinic Book of Home Remedies.* New York: Time Home Entertainment, Inc., 2010.

Halpin, Linda S., et al. "Guided Imagery in Cardiac Surgery." *Outcomes Management* 6, no. 3 (2002): 132–137.

Hanh, Thich Nhat. *You Are Here: Discovering the Magic of the Present Moment.* Boston: Shambhala Publications, Inc., 2009.

Hashim, Hairul Anuar, et al. "The Effects of Progressive Muscle Relaxation and Autogenic Relaxation on Young Soccer Players' Mood States." *Asian Journal of Sports Medicine* 2, no. 2 (2011): 99–105.

Hensrud, Donald D., medical editor in chief. *The Mayo Clinic Diet.* Cambridge, MA: Da Capo Press/Lifelong Books, 2010.

———. *The Mayo Clinic Diet Journal.* Cambridge, MA: Da Capo Press/Lifelong Books, 2010.

Hensrud, Donald D., et al. *The New Mayo Clinic Cookbook.* 2nd ed. New York: Oxmoor House Inc., an imprint of Time Inc. Books, 2012.

Holzel, Britta K., et al. "Mindfulness Practice Leads to Increases in Regional Brain Gray Matter Density." *Psychiatry Research* 19, no. 1 (2011): 36–43.

Hurt, Richard T., et al. "L-Arginine for the Treatment of Centrally Obese Subjects: A Pilot Study." *Journal of Dietary Supplements* 11, no. 1 (2014): 40–52.

Jahnke, Roger, et al. "A Comprehensive Review of Health Benefits of Qigong and Tai Chi." *American Journal of Health Promotion* 24, no. 6 (2010): e1–e25.

Kabat-Zinn, Jon. *Wherever You Go, There You Are.* New York: Hyperion, 1994.

Kalaaji, Amer N., et al. "Use of Complementary and Alternative Medicine by Patients Seen at the Dermatology Department of a Tertiary Care Center." *Complementary Therapies in Clinical Practice* 18, no. 1 (2012): 49–53.

Keller, Shelly R., et al. "Feasibility and Effectiveness of Massage Therapy for Symptom Relief in Cardiac Catheter Laboratory Staff: A Pilot Study." *Complementary Therapies in Clinical Practice* 18, no. 1 (2012): 4–9.

Kemper, Kathi J. *Authentic Healing: A Practical Guide for Caregivers.* Minneapolis, MN: Two Harbors Press, 2016.

Kiecolt-Glaser, Janice K., et al. "Hostile Marital Interactions, Proinflammatory Cytokine Production, and Wound Healing." *JAMA Psychiatry* 62, no. 12 (2005): 1377–1384.

Kim, Kun Hyung, et al. "Acupuncture for Lumbar Spinal Stenosis: A Systematic Review and Meta-Analysis." *Complementary Therapies in Medicine* 21 (2013): 535–556.

Kwekkeboom, Kristine L., et al. "Patients' Perceptions of the Effectiveness of Guided Imagery and Progressive Muscle Relaxation Interventions Used for Cancer Pain." *Complementary Therapies in Clinical Practice* 143, no. 3 (2008): 185–194.

Landry, Bradford W., et al. "Managing Chronic Pain in Children and Adolescents: A Clinical Review." *PM&R: The Journal of Injury, Function and Rehabilitation* 7 (11 Suppl) (Nov. 2015): S295–S315.

Lang, Susan S. "Americans' Circle of Confidantes Has Shrunk to Two People." *Cornell Chronicle*, Nov. 1, 2011. http://www.news.cornell.edu/stories/2011/11/americans-circle-confidantes-has-shrunk-two-people.

Litin, Scott, editor in chief. *Mayo Clinic Family Health Book.* 4th ed. Rochester, MN: Mayo Foundation for Medical Education and Research, 2009.

Liu, Lizhou, et al. "Acupuncture for Low Back Pain: An Overview of Systematic Reviews." *Evidence-Based Complementary and Alternative Medicine* 328196 (2015): 1–18.

Loewy, Joanne, et al. "The Effects of Music Therapy on Vital Signs, Feeding, and Sleep in Premature Infants." *Pediatrics* 131 (2013): 902–918.

Luders, Eileen, et al. "Forever Young(er): Potential Age-Defying Effects of Long-Term Meditation on Gray Matter Atrophy." *Frontiers in Psychology* 5 (2015): 1551.

Mallory, Molly J., et al. "Acupuncture in the Postoperative Setting for Breast Cancer Patients: A Feasibility Study." *The American Journal of Chinese Medicine* 43, no. 1 (2015): 45–56.

Martin, David P., et al. "Improvement in Fibromyalgia Symptoms with Acupuncture: Results of a Randomized Controlled Trial." *Mayo Clinic Proceedings* 81, no. 6 (2006): 749–757.

Maruta, Toshihiko, et al. "Optimism-Pessimism Assessed in the 1960s and Self-Reported Health Status 30 Years Later." *Mayo Clinic Proceedings* 77 (2002): 748–753.

Maruta, Toshihiko, et al. "Optimists vs. Pessimists: Survival Rate among Medical Patients over a 30-Year Period." *Mayo Clinic Proceedings* 75 (2000): 140–143.

Mayo Clinic Cancer Center. "A Creative Bedside Manner: Art, Music and Writing Offer Inspiration to Mayo Clinic Patients." *Together* 7, no. 1 (2007): 1.

Mayo Clinic. "Drugs and Supplements." http://www.mayoclinic.org/drugs-supplements. Accessed February 2, 2016.

McGarey, Gladys Taylor. *Physician within You.* Scottsdale, AZ: Inkwell Productions, 2000.

Moertl, Deddo, et al. "Dose-Dependent Effects of Omega-3-Polyunsaturated Fatty Acids on Systolic Left Ventricular Function, Endothelial Function, and Markers of Inflammation in Chronic Heart Failure of Nonischemic Origin: A Double-Blind, Placebo-Controlled, 3-Arm Study." *American Heart Journal* 161, no. 5 (2011): 915.e1–915.e9.

Morris, Martha Clare. "MIND Diet Associated with Reduced Incidence of Alzheimer's Disease." *Alzheimer's & Dementia* 11, no. 9 (2015): 1007–1014.

Mortenson, Svend A., et al. "The Effect of Coenzyme Q10 on Morbidity and Mortality in Chronic Heart Failure." *JACC: Heart Failure* 2, no. 6 (2014): 641–649.

National Center for Complementary and Integrative Health. "Herbs at a Glance." https://nccih.nih.gov/health/herbsataglance.htm. Accessed February 2, 2016.

———. "Spinal Manipulation's Effects May Go Beyond Those of Placebo or Expectation, Study Finds." October 27, 2013. https://nccih.nih.gov/research/results/spotlight/102713.

Natural Medicines Research Collaboration. "Spiritual Healing." https://naturalmedicines.therapeuticresearch.com. Accessed July 17, 2015.

NSF International. "What Is NSF Certification?" http://www.nsf.org/consumer-resources/what-is-nsf-certification/. Accessed February 2, 2016.

Ornish, Dean. *Dr. Dean Ornish's Program for Reversing Heart Disease.* New York: Random House Publishing Group, 1996.

Overcash, Janine, et al. "The Benefits of Medical Qigong in Patients with Cancer: A Descriptive Pilot Study." *Clinical Journal of Oncology Nursing* 17, no. 6 (2013): 654–658.

Pang, Ran, et al. "Complementary and Integrative Medicine at Mayo Clinic." *The American Journal of Chinese Medicine* 43, no. 8 (2015): 1503–1513.

Pavelká, Karel, et al. "Glucosamine Sulfate Use and Delay of Progression of Knee Osteoarthritis: A 3-Year, Randomized, Placebo-Controlled, Double-Blind Study." *Archives of Internal Medicine* 162, no. 18 (2002): 2113–2123.

Petersen, Ronald C., medical ed. *Mayo Clinic on Alzheimer's Disease.* Rochester, MN: Mayo Foundation for Medical Education and Research, 2013.

Pruthi, Sandhya, et al. "Value of Massage Therapy for Patients in a Breast Clinic." *Clinical Journal of Oncology Nursing* 13, no. 4 (2009): 422–425.

Pruthi, Sandhya, et al. "Vitamin E and Evening Primrose Oil for Management of Cyclical Castalgia: A Randomized Pilot Study." *Alternative Medicine Review: A Journal of Clinical Therapeutic* 15, no. 1 (2010): 59–67.

Rakel, D., and Kathy Sanders. *Project Health.* University of Wisconsin–Madison, 2013. https://itunes.apple.com/us/book/project-health/id634725466?mt=13.

Rausch, Sarah M., et al. "Complementary and Alternative Medicine: Use and Disclosure in Radiation Oncology Community Practice." *Supportive Care in Cancer* 19, no. 4 (2011): 521–529.

Reginster, Jean Yves, et al. "Long-Term Effects of Glucosamine Sulphate on Osteoarthritis Progression: A Randomised, Placebo-Controlled Clinical Trial." *The Lancet* 357, no. 9252 (2001): 251–256.

Rodgers, Nancy J., et al. "A Decade of Building Massage Therapy Services at an Academic Medical Center as Part of a Healing Enhancement Program." *Complementary Therapies in Clinical Practice* 21, no. 1 (2015): 52–56.

Salter, Shanah, and Sonya Brownie. "Treating Primary Insomnia: The Efficacy of Valerian and Hops." *Australian Family Physician* 39, no. 6 (2010): 433–437.

Scheufele, Peter M. "Effects of Progressive Muscle Relaxation and Classical Music on Measurements of Attention, Relaxation, and Stress Responses." *Journal of Behavioral Medicine* 23, no. 2 (2000): 207–228.

Schmidt, Michael A. *Beyond Antibiotics: Strategies for Living in a World of Emerging Infections and Antibiotic-Resistant Bacteria.* 3rd ed. Berkeley, CA: North Atlantic Books, 2009.

Schmidt, Michael A., and Jeffrey Bland. *Brain-Building Nutrition: How Dietary Fats and Oils Affect Mental, Physical, and Emotional Intelligence.* 3rd ed. Berkeley, CA: Frog Books, 2007.

Sharma, Varun, et al. "Bibliotherapy to Decrease Stress and Anxiety and Increase Resilience and Mindfulness: A Pilot Trial." *EXPLORE: The Journal of Science and Healing* 10, no. 4 (2014): 248–252.

Sierpina, Victor, and Steven Pratt. *The Healthy Gut Workbook: Whole-Body Healing for Heartburn, Ulcers, Constipation, IBS, Diverticulosis, and More.* Oakland, CA: New Harbinger Publications, Inc., 2010.

Song, Sunmi, et al. "The Role of Multiple Negative Social Relationships in Inflammatory Cytokine Responses to a Laboratory Stressor." *PeerJ* 3, no. e959 (2015): eCollection.

Sood, Amit. *Immerse: A 52-Week Course in Resilient Living.* Rochester, MN: Global Center for Resiliency and Wellbeing, 2016.

———. *The Mayo Clinic Guide to Stress-Free Living.* Cambridge, MA: Da Capo Press/Lifelong Books, 2013.

———. *The Mayo Clinic Handbook for Happiness: A 4-Step Plan for Resilient Living.* Cambridge, MA: Da Capo Press/Lifelong Books, 2015.

Sood, Amit, et al. "A Critical Review of Complementary Therapies for Cancer-Related Fatigue." *Integrative Cancer Therapies* 6, no. 1 (2007): 8–13.

Sood, Amit, et al. "A Randomized Clinical Trial of St. John's Wort for Smoking Cessation." *Journal of Alternative and Complementary Medicine* 16, no. 7 (2010): 761–767.

Sood, Amit, et al. "Stress Management and Resiliency Training (SMART) Program among Department of Radiology Faculty: A Pilot Randomized Clinical Trial." *EXPLORE: The Journal of Science and Healing* 10, no. 6 (2014): 358–363.

Suarez-Almazor, Maria. E., et al. "A Randomized Controlled Trial of Acupuncture for Osteoarthritis of the Knee: Effects of Patient-Provider Communication." *Arthritis Care & Research* 62, no. 9 (2010): 1229–1236.

Takahashi, Toku. "Mechanism of Acupuncture on Neuromodulation in the Gut—A Review." *Neuromodulation: Technology at the Neural Interface* 14 (2011): 8–12.

Terjestam, Yvonne, et al. "Effects of Scheduled Qigong Exercise on Pupils' Well-Being, Self-Image, Distress, and Stress." *The Journal of Alternative and Complementary Medicine* 16, no. 9 (2010): 939–944.

Texas A&M University. "A Risky Soaking: Study Shows Whirlpool Water Can Be Dangerous." January 23, 2006. http://www.science.tamu.edu/news/story.php?story_ID=493.

Thicke, Lori A., et al. "Acupuncture for Treatment of Noncyclic Breast Pain: A Pilot Study." *The American Journal of Chinese Medicine* 39, no. 6 (2011): 1117–1129.

Thomley, Barbara S., et al. "Effects of a Brief, Comprehensive, Yoga-Based Program on Quality of Life and Biometric Measures in an Employee Population: A Pilot Study." *Explore (NY)* 7, no. 1 (2011): 27–29.

Thompson, Michael A., et al. "Dietary Supplement S-Adenosyl-L-Methionine (AdoMet) Effects on Plasma Homocysteine Levels in Healthy Human Subjects: A Double-Blind, Placebo-Controlled, Randomized Clinical Trial." *Journal of Alternative and Complementary Medicine* 15, no. 5 (2009): 523–529.

Tsang, Hector W. H., and Kelvin M. T. Fung. "A Review on Neurobiological and Psychological Mechanisms Underlying the Anti-Depressive Effect of Qigong Exercise." *Journal of Health Psychology* 13, no. 7 (2008): 857–863.

U.S. Department of Health and Human Services, National Institutes of Health, Eunice Kennedy Shriver National Institute of Child Health and Human Development. "Neuroplasticity." https://www.nichd.nih.gov/about/overview/50th/discoveries/Pages/neuroplasticity.aspx. Accessed June 24, 2015.

"Understanding Acupuncture: Time to Try It?" *NIH News in Health.* February 2011. http://newsinhealth.nih.gov/issue/feb2011/Feature1.

United States Pharmacopeia. "USP Verification Services." http://www.usp.org/usp-verification-services. Accessed February 2, 2016.

Vincent, Ann, et al. "External Qigong for Chronic Pain." *The American Journal of Chinese Medicine* 38, no. 4 (2010): 695–703.

Vincent, Ann, et al. "Utilisation of Acupuncture at an Academic Medical Centre." *Acupuncture in Medicine* 28, no. 4 (2010): 189–190.

Wahner-Roedler, Dietlind L., et al. "Development of a Complementary and Alternative Medicine Programme at an Academic Medical Centre." *Evidence-Based Integrative Medicine* 2, no. 1 (2005): 9–12.

Wahner-Roedler, Dietlind L., et al. "Dietary Soy Supplement on Fibromyalgia Symptoms: A Randomized, Double-Blind, Placebo-Controlled, Early Phase Trial." *Evidence-Based Complementary and Alternative Medicine* 2011 (2011): Epub June 23, 2011.

Wahner-Roedler, Dietlind L., et al. "Physicians' Attitudes toward Complementary and Alternative Medicine and Their Knowledge of Specific Therapies: A Survey at an Academic Medical Center. *Evidence-Based Complementary and Alternative Medicine* 3, no. 4 (2006): 495–501.

Wahner-Roedler, Dietlind L., et al. "Physicians' Attitudes toward Complementary and Alternative Medicine and Their Knowledge of

Specific Therapies: 8-Year Follow-Up at an Academic Medical Center." *Complementary Therapies in Clinical Practice* 20, no. 1 (2014): 54–60.

Wahner-Roedler, Dietlind L., et al. "The Effect of Grape Seed Extract on Estrogen Levels of Postmenopausal Women: A Pilot Study." *Journal of Dietary Supplements* 11, no. 2 (2014): 184–197.

Wahner-Roedler, Dietlind L., et al. "Use of Complementary and Alternative Medical Therapies by Patients Referred to a Fibromyalgia Treatment Program at a Tertiary Care Center." *Mayo Clinic Proceedings* 80, no. 1 (2005): 55–60.

Waller, Elisabeth, et al. "Unresolved Trauma in Fibromyalgia: A Cross-Sectional Study." *Journal of Health Psychology* (2015): 1–9.

Wang, Chong-Wen, et al. "Managing Stress and Anxiety through Qigong Exercise in Healthy Adults: A Systematic Review and Meta-Analysis of Randomized Controlled Trials." B*MC Complementary and Alternative Medicine* 14 (2014): 8–17.

Weil, Andrew. *8 Weeks to Optimum Health.* New York: Ballantine Books, 2007.

Wentworth, Laura J., et al. "Massage Therapy Reduces Tension, Anxiety, and Pain in Patients Awaiting Invasive Cardiovascular Procedures." *Progress in Cardiovascular Nursing* 24, no. 4 (2009): 155–161.

Wolever, Ruth Q., and Beth Reardon, with Tania Hannan. *The Mindful Diet: How to Transform Your Relationship with Food for Lasting Weight Loss and Vibrant Health.* New York: Scribner, An Imprint of Simon & Schuster, Inc., 2015.

World Health Organization. "Spending on Health: A Global Overview." http://www.who.int/mediacentre/factsheets/fs319/en/. Accessed June 9, 2015.

Xin, Wei, et al. "Effects of Fish Oil Supplementation on Cardiac Function in Chronic Heart Failure: A Meta-Analysis of Randomized Controlled Trials." *Heart* 98 (2012): 1620–1625.

Yoo, Hee J., et al. "Efficacy of Progressive Muscle Relaxation Training and Guided Imagery in Reducing Chemotherapy Side Effects in Patients with Breast Cancer and in Improving Their Quality of Life." *Support Care Cancer* 13 (2005): 826–833.

Zhang, Tao, et al. "Efficacy of Acupuncture for Chronic Constipation: A Systematic Review." *The American Journal of Chinese Medicine* 41, no. 4 (2013): 717–742.

Zick, Susanna M., et al. "Hawthorn Extract Randomized Blinded Chronic Heart Failure (HERB CHF) Trial." *European Journal of Heart Failure* 11, no. 10 (2009): 990–999.

Image Credits

Page No.

4	© cyano66/iStock/Thinkstock.
9	© FogStock/FogStock Collection/Thinkstock.
10	© Mike Powell/DigitalVision/Thinkstock.
26	© Yuliya Gontar/Shutterstock.
31	© LADYING/Shutterstock.
47	© Kerdkanno/Shutterstock.
50	© fStop Images GmbH/Shutterstock.
71	© Ania Klara/Shutterstock.
74	© Kittibowornphatnon/Shutterstock.
91	© GlebStock/Shutterstock.
97	© Andrea Danti/Shutterstock.
113	© Kuznetcov_Konstantin/Shutterstock.
116	© Image Point Fr/Shutterstock.
120	© Pavel L Photo and Video/Shutterstock.
137	© Dragon Images/Shutterstock.
140	© Luna Vandoorne/Shutterstock.
143	© Darren Baker/Shutterstock.
158	© wavebreakmedia/Shutterstock.
164	© Markus Gann/Shutterstock.
185	© Zai Aragon/Shutterstock.
187	© wckiw/Shutterstock.
188	© Malysh A/Shutterstock.
204	© fotohunter/Shutterstock.
210	© fotohunter/Shutterstock.
226	© wavebreakmedia/Shutterstock.
231	© gajdamak/Shutterstock.
250	© ORLIO/Shutterstock.
253	© Andor Bujdoso/Shutterstock.
256	© pio3/Shutterstock.